MAGNETIC RESONANCE IMAGING IN FOODS

MAGNETIC RESONANCE IMAGING IN FOODS

MICHAEL J. McCARTHY

CHAPMAN & HALL
New York • London

First published in 1994 by
Chapman & Hall
One Penn Plaza
New York, NY 10119

Published in Great Britain by
Chapman & Hall
2–6 Boundary Row
London SE1 8HN

Printed in the United States of America

Library of Congress Cataloging in Publication Data

McCarthy, Michael J. (Michael John), 1957–
Magnetic resonance imaging in foods / Michael J. McCarthy.
p. cm.
Includes bibliographical references and index.
ISBN 0-412-98811-9
1. Food—Analysis. 2. Magnetic resonance imaging. I. Title.
TX542.M33 1994
664′.07—dc20 93-48653
CIP

British Library Cataloguing in Publication Data available

Please send your order for this or any other Chapman & Hall book to **Chapman & Hall, 29 West 35th Street, New York, NY 10001, Attn: Customer Service Department.** You may also call our Order Department at 1-212-244-3336 or fax your purchase order to 1-800-248-4724.

For a complete listing of Chapman & Hall's titles, send your request to **Chapman & Hall, Dept. BC, One Penn Plaza, New York, NY 10119.**

Table of Contents

Preface ix

1. Introduction to Magnetic Resonance Imaging (MRI) 1
  - Introduction to Magnetic Resonance 3
    - Definition of Magnetic Resonance 3
      - Nuclear Magnetic Resonance (NMR) 3
      - Electron Spin Resonance (ESR) 4
    - Characteristics of NMR 4
    - History of NMR 4
    - NMR Equipment and Experiments 5
      - Components of an NMR Spectrometer 5
      - Pulse Sequences 7
      - Low-resolution NMR 7
      - High-resolution NMR 10
      - Two-dimensional NMR 10
      - Pulsed Field Gradient Experiments 10
      - MRI Techniques 11
        - Property-weighted Imaging 14
        - Chemical Shift Imaging 14
        - Microscopy 14
  - Applications and Impact of MRI on Food Research 14
    - Food Stability and Structure 14
      - Foams 14
      - Emulsions 16
      - Gels 17
      - Moisture Migration 17
        - Dehydration/Rehydration 17
        - Storage 18
      - Rheology 19
      - Phase Changes 19

Freezing 19
Lipid Crystallization 20
Capabilities and Limitations of MRI 21
Density Imaging 22
Temperature Range 22
Moisture Content Range 22
Diffusion/Flow Imaging 22
Diffusivity Range 22
Velocity Range 22
Temperature Imaging 22
Structural Imaging 23
Voids 23
Water and/or Lipid 23
Chemical Shift Effect 24
Magnetic Susceptibility Effect 25
Image Resolution 26
Spatial 26
Temporal 26
References 27

2. Fundamental Principles of Magnetic Resonance Imaging 30
Quantum Mechanical Description NMR 30
Bloch Model of NMR 31
Characteristics of Physical System for which Bloch Model is Correct 31
Relaxation Effects 32
Pulse Sequences 33
One-pulse 33
Spin Echo 34
Stimulated Echo 37
Magnetic Resonance Imaging 37
Slice Selection 38
Phase Encoding 39
Frequency Encoding 40
Fourier Imaging 40
Echo-planar Imaging 41
Projection Reconstruction 41
Interpretation of Spin-warp Imaging Signals 41
Information Content of NMR Image 41
Comparison of NMR Image Data to Theoretical Models 42
Basis of Theoretical Models 42
Mathematical Basis for Comparison 43
References 44

3. Measurement of Food Structure and Component Functionality 45
Structure Measurement 45
Experimental Setup 45

Probe 45
Sample Container 46
Process Equipment 47
Spectrometer Setup 49
Shielded Gradients 50
Analysis of NMR Signal 51
Phase Volume Measurements/Concentrations 51
Dynamics 52
Flow Measurements 52
Examples of Food Structure Measurement 54
Foams 54
Experimental Procedures and Data Analysis 54
Phase Volume 54
Liquid Drainage 56
Collapse 56
Relaxation Effects 56
Additional Applications 56
Emulsions 57
Experimental Procedures and Data Analysis 57
Phase Volume 57
Droplet Size Distribution 60
Additional Applications 61
Suspensions 62
Experimental Procedures and Data Analysis 62
Velocity Measurements 62
Rheological Information 65
Additional Applications 67
References 67

4. Moisture and Lipid Distributions 70
Saturation Measurements 70
Experimental Setup 70
Probe 70
Sample Container 71
Spectrometer Setup 72
Analysis of NMR Signal 72
Spin-warp Imaging 72
Relaxation Effects 72
Temperature Effects 74
Quantification of Water and Lipid Signals 74
Relationship of Signal Intensities to Concentration Values 75
Moisture Saturation Measurements 78
Drying of Agricultural Products 78
Apples 78
Potatoes 78
Corn 80
Gels 80

Drying of Porous Media 80
Use of Zero-, One-, and Two-dimensional Data 80
Film Thickness Measurements 82
Lipid Saturation Measurements 83
Medical 84
Animal 84
Processed Food 84
References 86

5. Phase Transitions 88
Quantification 88
Experimental Setup 88
Probe 88
Sample Container 88
Process Equipment 89
Spectrometer Setup 89
Analysis of NMR Signal 90
Relaxation Effects 90
Temperature Effects 91
Phase Volume Changes 94
MRI versus Localized Spectroscopy 94
Lipid Crystallization 94
Phase Volume 94
Low-resolution 96
NMR Imaging 97
Differential Scanning Calorimetry (DSC) 97
Freezing of Water 97
Food Systems 97
Comparison of MRI Data to Mathematical Models 98
State of Water in Frozen Systems 98
References 99

6. Future Trends and Conclusions 101
Future Trends 101
Analytical Methods 102
Process Control Sensor 102
Conclusions 103
References 104

Preface

Nuclear magnetic resonance imaging is one of several new experimental techniques which have recently been applied to food systems. NMR in general and nuclear magnetic resonance imaging are powerful probes of the microscopic and macroscopic changes occurring in foods during processing, storage and utilization. The training that food scientists and food engineers have received in the past has often omitted specific courses in physical chemistry that form the theoretical and practical foundation necessary to fully utilized magnetic resonance experimental techniques.

The goal of *Magnetic Resonance Imaging in Foods* is to introduce food scientists and food engineers to magnetic resonance imaging and provide a basis for further study. As such the book begins with two chapters of an introductory nature. The first chapter introduces magnetic resonance phenomena, NMR in general, and MRI in detail. Particular emphasis is given to the limitations and typical ranges available for studying particular phenomena, for example, the range of diffusivities that can be studied using commercial grade NMR equipment. Chapter 2 gives a brief introduction to the classical physical model of NMR first introduced by Felix Bloch in 1946 and aspects important to the interpretation of MRI data. This chapter is provided for the researchers and students interested in more details of the basic theory. Chapter 2 can be skipped by those individuals not requiring more information on the basic theory of NMR. The next several chapters of the book are on applications of MRI to food systems.

Each chapter on applications begins with a section of information about the specific type of experiment to be discussed. These beginning sections are for individuals who are just starting to use MRI in food research. As such, the sections include information not typically discussed in the research literature, for example, the steps required to build a successful process simulation for use in a MRI spectrometer. Those readers interested in the results available from specific experiments can proceed directly to the relevant sections.

No attempt has been made to include all of the literature relevant to magnetic resonance imaging of foods. This book is intended as an introduction and starting place for researchers, students, and managers.

Acknowledgments

Students and research scientists working in my laboratory have been particularly helpful in reviewing sections, assisting with illustrations, and providing valuable comments. I am particularly grateful to Professor Robert Kauten and Professor J. Bruce German for their support. I am grateful to Carole Hinkle who provided technical editing for the major portion of this book. Special thanks to my wife and co-worker, Professor Kathryn L. McCarthy, for encouragement and assistance.

1

Introduction to Magnetic Resonance Imaging (MRI)

Throughout history, much time and attention have been spent on quantifying and predicting the changes in foods during processing and storage. Despite much research in this area, there is still a considerable lack of fundamental information concerning the physiochemical changes and transport phenomena occurring in foods. One of the major impediments to acquiring this knowledge has been the inability to measure or probe food systems without altering the phenomena being measured. Consider, for example, a classical approach to measuring the temperature of a particle flowing in a fluid during heat exchange. If a thermocouple is placed in the food particle, the flow characteristics of the particle are altered, and subsequently the heat transfer is altered. The measured value of the temperature, therefore, becomes more or less dependent on the technique of measurement. Another example is the rheological characterization of a fibrous suspension such as tomato paste. If a typical rheometer is used to characterize the fluid, this measurement assumes a well-defined flow profile and a well-mixed system in order to provide accurate information. However, considerable recent information indicates that particles in this type of flow may migrate. It is difficult to determine whether the measured information characterizes the actual fluid or some newly structured fluid/particle system which may or may not reflect the conditions in the actual process environment. During the past 10 years, food scientists have begun to address some of these issues by using the technique of magnetic resonance imaging (MRI).

Magnetic resonance images of the velocity profile of tomato juice and the internal structure of Swiss cheese are shown in Figure 1.1. For the tomato juice flow image, the signal intensity is related to the amount of fluid flowing at a given velocity at a specific radial position in the pipe; the lighter the gray scale, the greater the density. This image was obtained for tomato juice flowing in a 1″ inner diameter pipe and reflects the conditions similar to those found in a tomato processing facility. The image of the Swiss cheese gives an indication

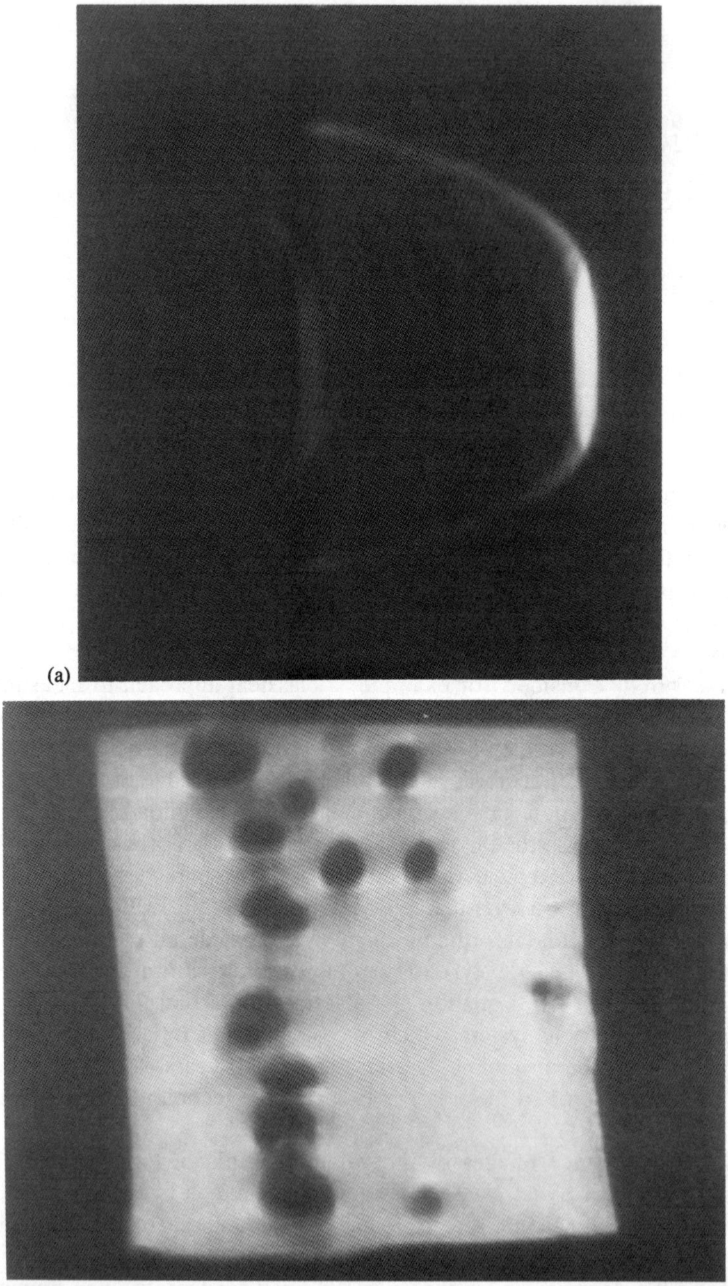

(a)
(b)

Figure 1.1. (a) Magnetic resonance images of the fluid velocity profile of tomato juice in a pipe and (b) the hydrogen nuclei density in a plane through a block of Swiss cheese.

of the total amount of both water and oil signals at each spatial position. As in the flow image, gray scale intensity is proportional to density. The image of the Swiss cheese provides information on the structure and quality of the product.

This book will provide an introduction to magnetic resonance, an overview of many current applications of MRI in food research, and a series of strategies for application of these techniques. Applications that are emphasized include food structure measurement, moisture and lipid distributions, and phase transitions.

Introduction to Magnetic Resonance

Definition of Magnetic Resonance

Magnetic resonance is a phenomenon that occurs between atomic particles and an external magnetic field. The atomic particles responsible for this interaction are the electrons and the nucleus. The interaction between the atomic particles and the external magnetic field is similar to what happens when iron filings are placed near a bar magnet. The filings become oriented and a magnetic field is induced in the metal. However, unlike the filings, the physical orientation of the atomic particles is not altered. At most common magnetic field strengths only the magnetic moment of the atomic particles is influenced.

The phenomenon of resonance is observed in these systems because they absorb and emit energy at specific frequencies. The specific frequency depends on the individual atomic particle and the strength of the applied magnetic field.

Nuclear Magnetic Resonance (NMR)

When the atomic particle is a nucleus the phenomenon is termed *nuclear magnetic resonance*. Not all nuclei exhibit magnetic resonance. A nucleus has a magnetic moment only if the spin angular moment is non-zero. Common nuclei with magnetic moments include ^{1}H, ^{31}P, ^{15}N, ^{23}Na; nuclei without magnetic moments include ^{12}C and ^{16}O.

NMR is frequently referred to simply as magnetic resonance, especially in medical applications. The term *nuclear* is omitted so that patients will not confuse this technique with nuclear medical procedures that use radioactive materials. NMR is generally a very safe experimental procedure and does not harm or alter the environment, the operator, or the sample.

NMR is a particularly useful spectroscopy because the signal emitted from a sample is sensitive to the number of nuclei, to the chemical and electronic surroundings of the nuclei at the molecular level, and to the diffusion or flow of the nuclei. This sensitivity to a range of sample characteristics is responsible for the wide use of NMR in chemistry, biochemistry, biotechnology, petrophysics, plastics, engineering, building materials, consumer products, medicine, and food technology. The applications of NMR range from routine moisture and fat content measurements in food production facilities to the determination of molecular structure of proteins and the dynamics of water in biological systems.

Electron Spin Resonance (ESR)

The second type of magnetic resonance is called *electron spin resonance* (ESR) or *electron paramagnetic resonance*. The terms refer to the interaction between an electron's magnetic moment and an external applied magnetic field. As is the case with nuclei, not all electrons in atoms exhibit magnetic resonance. Only unpaired electrons give rise to an ESR signal or spectra. Hence, ESR spectra are most often from ions, radicals, and short-lifetime intermediates. ESR is typically used to study the structure of crystals, the influence of radiation on materials, organic reactions, and reactions in biological materials.

Characteristics of NMR

Placement of a sample of water in a magnetic field will result in the orientation of the ^{1}H nuclear magnetic moments. The orientation is not instantaneous but takes place exponentially over several seconds. The ^{1}H nuclear magnetic moments achieve an equilibrium state. In order to displace the system from equilibrium, energy is added to the sample of water by applying an additional magnetic field for a period of time (on the order of tens of microseconds). The added energy perturbs the nuclear magnetic moments from equilibrium. Since the energy is added by use of a magnetic field and since the amounts of energy are extremely small, this spectroscopy is both noninvasive and nondestructive.

The emitted electromagnetic radiation can be made proportional to the nuclei number density, chemical structure, molecular or atomic diffusion coefficients, reaction rates, chemical exchange, and other phenomena. By acquisition of several sets of emissions over time, transient phenomena such as drying, freezing, lipid migration, and volumetric changes can be followed and quantified.

History of NMR

The initial successful nuclear magnetic resonance experiments were performed in the laboratories of F. Bloch and E. Purcell. These experiments were conducted independently and published in 1946 (Bloch 1946). The development of NMR spectroscopy proceeded quickly as many different nuclei were studied and different effects discovered.

Use of NMR in analysis of chemical and biochemical molecules is an essential tool for research. Advances in fields other than food technology have provided NMR spectroscopists with the ability to dramatically improve both experiments and data analysis. In the area of magnet design, advances enabling very high magnetic field systems have allowed NMR to be used to study fine details of molecular structure. Advances in computer technology coupled with digital fast

Fourier transforms have allowed for the development of multidimensional NMR methods (described in the next section). Occurring simultaneously with the development of multidimensional NMR was the technique of generating images of the internal structure of materials with NMR (Lauterbur 1973; Mansfield & Grannell 1973). Called NMR imaging or magnetic resonance imaging, this technique has been primarily applied in biomedical research and as a radiological diagnostic tool. One can read almost daily about professional athletes undergoing MRI scans in order to determine the extent of their injuries.

Extensive application of MRI to study the structure and dynamics of nonbiological materials and biological materials not directly related to medical research was sporadic until the early 1980's. Many early researchers mentioned that this technique could revolutionize food research. For example, Morris (1986) suggested that MRI be used in the study of seed germination and determination of the optimum time for processing seeds. Mansfield and Morris (1982) suggested studies of moisture migration in foods and detection of ripeness and decay in fruits and vegetables. Since 1980, the technique has become an important new tool for quantifying transport phenomena, kinetics, structural defects, and dynamics of multiphase systems (Maneval et al. 1992). Multiphase systems include the flow of suspensions, quality defects in plastics, water relationships in foods, moisture transport in ceramics, and temperature measurements in gels and tissues; quality attributes of fruits, vegetables, and cheeses have also been studied using MRI (McCarthy et al. 1991; McCarthy & Kauten 1990; Schmidt & Lai 1991).

NMR Equipment and Experiments

NMR spectroscopy can be subdivided into a number of different types of experiments. The classifications useful for most food analysis applications are low-resolution, high-resolution, two-dimensional techniques, spatially localized spectra, pulsed field gradient experiments, and magnetic resonance images, including chemical shift imaging, property-weighted imaging, and microscopy. Distinctions between these techniques result from both differences in hardware (e.g., magnet strength, magnetic field homogeneity) and in experimental design of the pulse sequence. A pulse sequence is a series of excitations and time delays applied to the sample through the NMR spectrometer. Pulse sequences are varied to weight the information content of an experiment; for example, in order to measure the mobility of water, a spin echo pulse sequence is used that requires multiple pulse excitations.

Components of an NMR Spectrometer

The basic components of an NMR spectrometer are detailed in Figure 1.2. The range of magnetic field strengths is normally from 0.1 to 10 tesla. The shape and size of magnets can vary dramatically. Small magnets are available in a

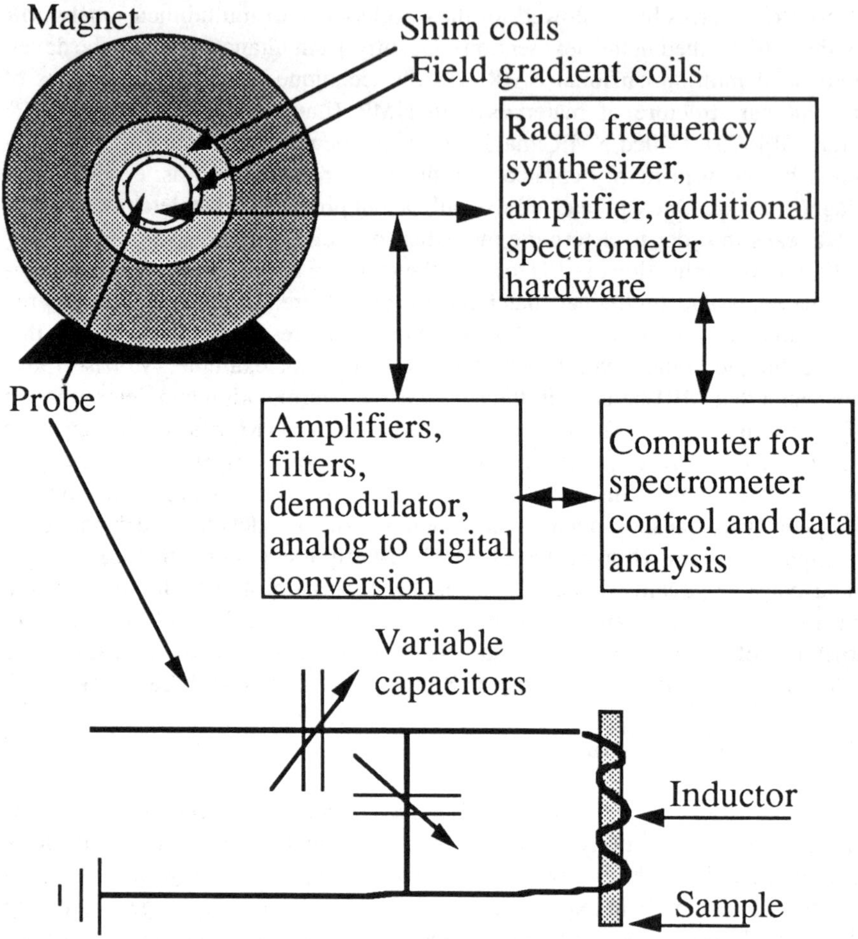

Figure 1.2. Essential components of magnetic resonance imaging spectrometer.

bench top enclosure that require only half a meter of space. Whole-body medical imaging systems require a specially designed room with a high ceiling and significantly reduced amounts of steel.

Within the magnet are various electromagnetic coils called shim coils. Electrical current is adjusted in these shim coils in order to homogenize the static magnetic field across the sample. For an MRI spectrometer, specially designed magnetic field gradient coils are incorporated into the bore of the magnet. These field gradient coils are usually designed to generate linear variations in the magnetic field across the sample region. Applying linear magnetic field gradients alters the homogeneity of the field in a predictable fashion and is used to spatially encode the NMR signal.

To couple the sample to the spectrometer, a probe or coil is placed around the sample and then the probe and sample are placed as a unit inside the magnet. The electrical components in the probe are capacitors and an inductor. The capacitors are used to adjust the frequency and impedance of the circuit for maximum efficiency. The inductor is used to transmit the radio frequency (RF) energy and to pick up the induced NMR signal from the sample; hence, the sample is located within the inductor coil. There are many different designs for probes. Shown in Figure 1.2 is a simple solenoid design. Other designs include surface coils in which the inductor is just a circular loop of wire placed under the sample or a birdcage design which is a tunnel-shape placed around the sample.

RF energy used to displace the system from equilibrium is supplied by a frequency synthesizer. The RF signal is amplified and pulsed into the probe in short bursts (usually 10 μs to 2ms long). The excitation pulses vary in power from 100 W to several kW.

A signal is recorded from the sample immediately after the pulse. The signal strength is very weak, generally in the micro- to millivolt range. This signal is amplified, filtered, demodulated, and digitized for storage and display. The process of demodulation occurs when the signal from the sample is mixed with the original excitation frequency. The difference in frequencies is the NMR time domain signal. This intensity versus time signal is usually Fourier transformed prior to analysis which produces an intensity versus frequency plot called the NMR spectrum (Figure 1.3).

Pulse Sequences

A pulse sequence is a set of instructions dictating the order of events in an NMR experiment. A timing diagram for a spin-warp MRI pulse sequence, shown in Figure 1.4, includes RF pulses, field gradient pulses, and data acquisition windows. Most MRI pulse sequences can be interpreted in terms of a classical two-dimensional NMR experiment having three separate sections: preparation, evolution, and detection (a mixing period needs to be included if multiple quantum transitions are desired). During the preparation period, the nuclear spin system is displaced from equilibrium. The evolution period allows the evolution of the nuclear spin system to be influenced by a parameter that is to be measured. In Figure 1.4, the phase of the NMR signal is altered to encode spatial positions along the direction of a gradient. The detection period is the time during which the NMR signal is recorded.

Low-resolution NMR

Low-resolution experiments are run on spectrometers with low magnetic field strength, usually below 1 tesla. The time domain signal from a low-resolution NMR system is shown in Figure 1.5. Discrimination of different components

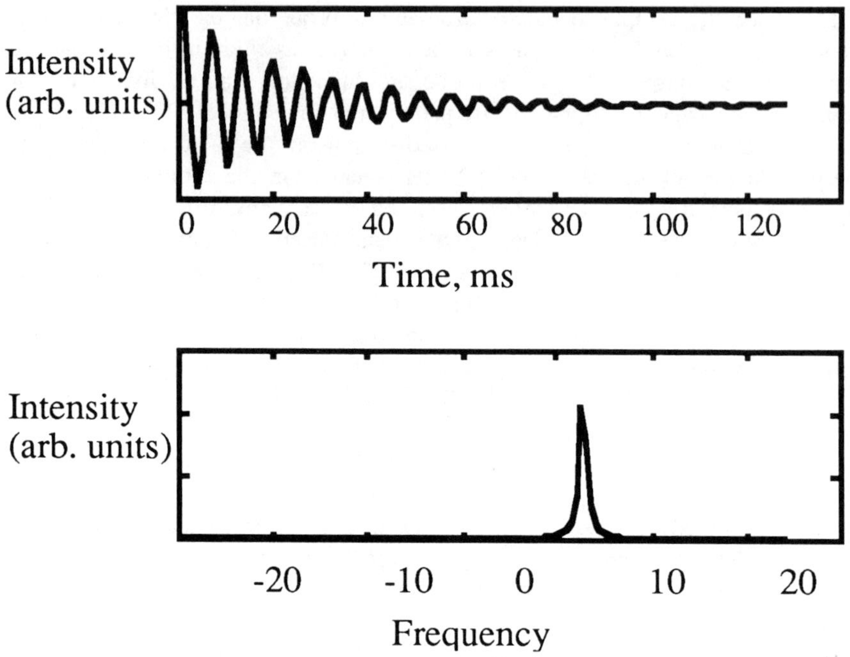

Figure 1.3. Simulation of real part of free induction decay and real part of Fourier transform spectrum.

based on analysis of the frequency content of the NMR data is generally not possible with low-resolution systems which are used to measure relaxation times of the sample. The two relaxation times are the spin-lattice relaxation time and the spin-spin relaxation time.

Relaxation time measurements provide information on the interactions of the nuclear magnetic moments within the sample. Spin-lattice relaxation characterizes the rate of energy exchange between the nuclear magnetic moments and the rest of the sample (the lattice). Spin-spin relaxation describes the loss of coherence among the nuclear magnetic moments and is therefore an entropic effect (Morris 1986).

The NMR signal from low-resolution experiments is usually analyzed in the time domain to provide information on moisture content, fat content, or solids content. These types of NMR systems are normally small and can be placed on top of a wooden laboratory bench. Several low-resolution systems have been adapted for on-line control of fat and moisture and the tempering of wheat (Schmidt 1991). Low-resolution NMR could be adapted for use in control of many food processes such as mixing ground meat and sorting fresh fruits and vegetables.

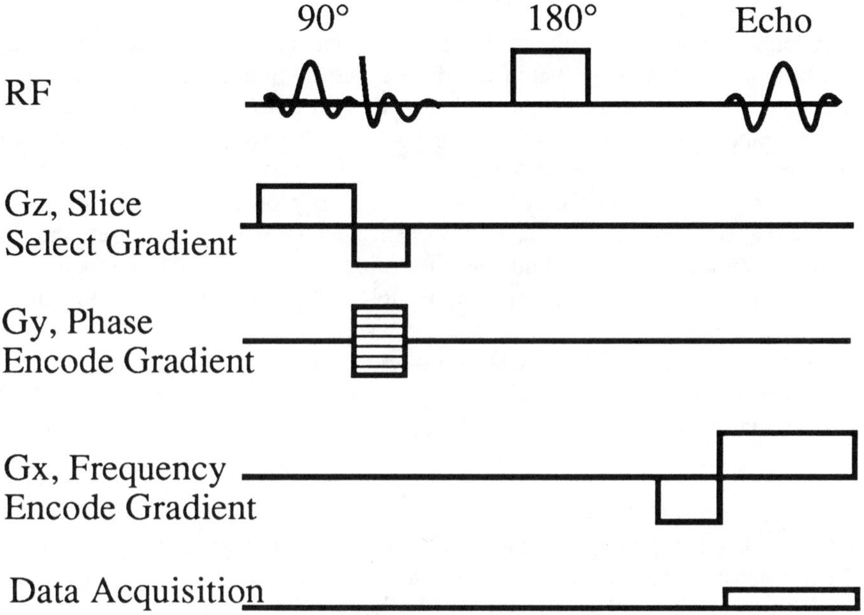

Figure 1.4. Pulse sequence timing diagram for standard spin-warp MRI imaging experiment.

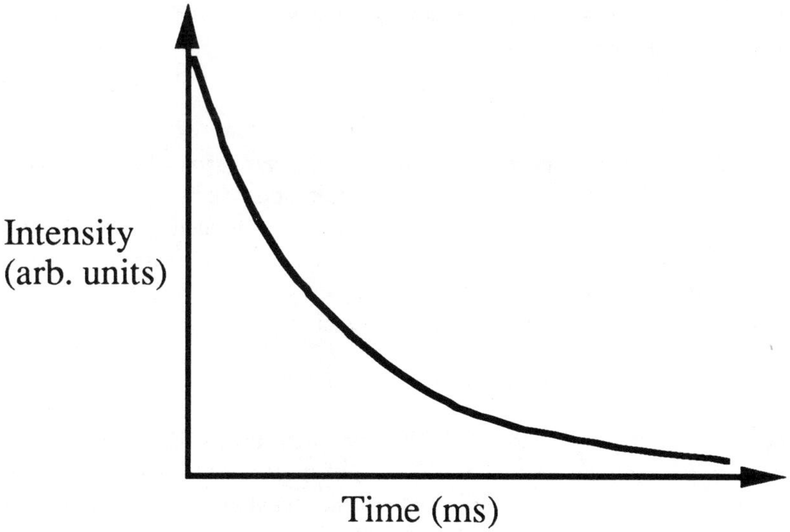

Figure 1.5. Time domain signal from sample in low-resolution NMR spectrometer.

High-resolution NMR

A high-resolution experiment differentiates between nuclei in one molecular environment and another based on differences in frequency of excitation or resonance. Figure 1.6 is a typical high-resolution NMR spectrum. Differences in the frequency of excitation result from variations in structure and local chemical environment for each nucleus.

The frequency of excitation for each nucleus is proportional to the magnetic field at the spatial position of that nucleus. The nuclei in a molecule can experience slightly different magnetic fields because other nuclear magnetic moments add or subtract from the external magnetic field. The resulting shift in resonant frequencies is referred to as the chemical shift and is expressed in parts per million from the frequency of a standard reference. The differences in chemical shift arise from different local chemical and electronic environments. This effect can be quantified by

$$\nu = \gamma \, \mathrm{Bo} \, (1 - \sigma)/2\pi \qquad [1.1]$$

where σ is the shielding constant, and γ is the magnetogryic ratio, a constant for a given nucleus. Values of the shielding constant range between 10^{-3} and 10^{-6} for most nuclei (Gadian 1982).

High-resolution NMR is used to identify chemical compounds, determine if a food has been irradiated, characterize the structure of a macromolecule, and to measure packing and polymorphism in polymers. Results from high-resolution NMR experiments and two-dimensional NMR experiments are utilized with molecular modeling software to determine the solution structure of small- to medium-size macromolecules.

Two-dimensional NMR

Many high-resolution spectra are difficult to analyze; a two-dimensional NMR spectrum is needed for an improved interpretation. Such a two-dimensional spectrum consists of a function with two independent frequency variables (Ernst, Bodenhausen & Wokaun 1987). Figure 1.7 is the two-dimensional spectra of sucrose. Common experiments include such independent variable pairs as chemical shift vs. scalar couplings and chemical shift vs. dipolar couplings.

Pulsed Field Gradient Experiments

The decay of the signal in an NMR experiment based on a spin echo pulse sequence can be influenced by the diffusion of molecules to which the observed nuclei are attached. The additional decay of the signal arises from the movement of the nuclei through magnetic field gradients found within the internal structure of the sample or applied by the experimenter to enhance the effect. A pulsed

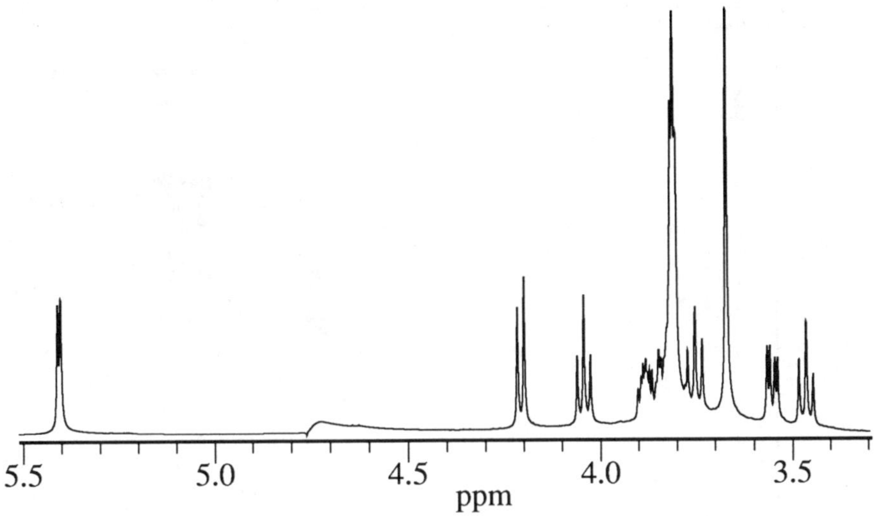

Figure 1.6. A high-resolution NMR spectrum of hydrogen in sucrose.

field gradient experiment utilizes two short field gradient pulses before and after the 180° pulse in a spin echo experiment. Typically the time between the pulses or the gradient strength is changed to vary the magnitude of the additional decay. Analysis of a plot of the amplitude decay vs. the parameter varied yields an estimate of the self-diffusion coefficient of the molecule to which the nuclei are attached, as shown in Figure 1.8. This is an excellent method to measure the self-diffusion coefficient of a molecule. By making analogies to diffraction experiments, self-diffusion data has recently been used to measure material structure (Barrall, Frydman & Chingas 1992; Callaghan 1991).

MRI Techniques

Magnetic resonance imaging is an NMR technique which provides spatial localization of the NMR signals from a sample. Thus, the signals from many neighboring spatial locations can be used to generate an image of nuclei density or some other property. MRI is based on degrading the homogeneity of the external magnetic field in a predictable pattern. This results in a known frequency variation across the sample. The frequency variation is usually achieved by the application of a linear magnetic field gradient. If the effects of the shielding constant are ignored, the frequency of excitation and detection for an NMR experiment is given by the Larmor equation (Abragam 1961):

$$\nu = \gamma \, Bo/2\pi \qquad [1.2]$$

By applying a linear field gradient in the z direction, the frequency becomes a function of position (Mansfield & Morris 1982):

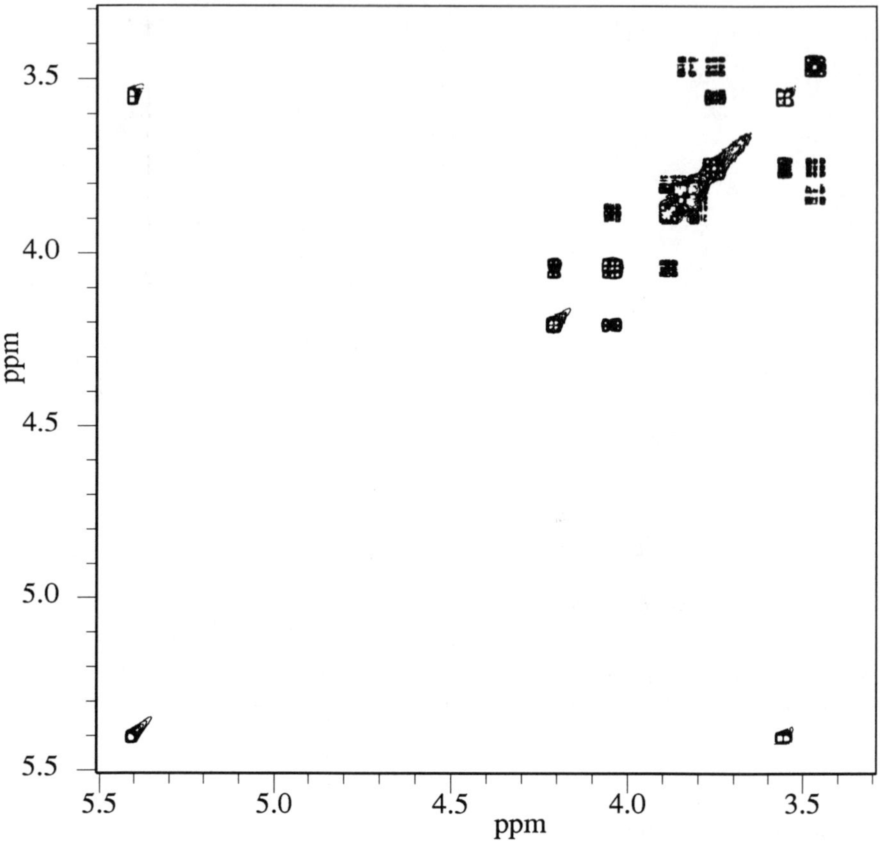

Figure 1.7. A two-dimensional NMR spectrum of hydrogen in sucrose.

$$\nu(z) = \gamma\,(Bo + G_z\,z)/2\pi \qquad [1.3]$$

where G_z is the strength of the magnetic field gradient in the z direction and z is spatial position. The effect of this gradient on an NMR spectrum is detailed in Figure 1.9.

MRI techniques can be further subdivided into point, line, plane, and three-dimensional spatial images. However, it is important to note that the signal for each voxel in an image is actually the weighted signal from a three-dimensional volume element. Therefore, the signal from a point experiment might be from a 0.5 mm^3 shaped volume in the center of an object. Point images or localized spectra are high-resolution NMR spectra recorded from a specific location within an object. A line image is really the extension of a point image along one axis and is thus a series of small volumes next to each other. A line image differs from a localized spectra in that usually no chemical shift information is retained.

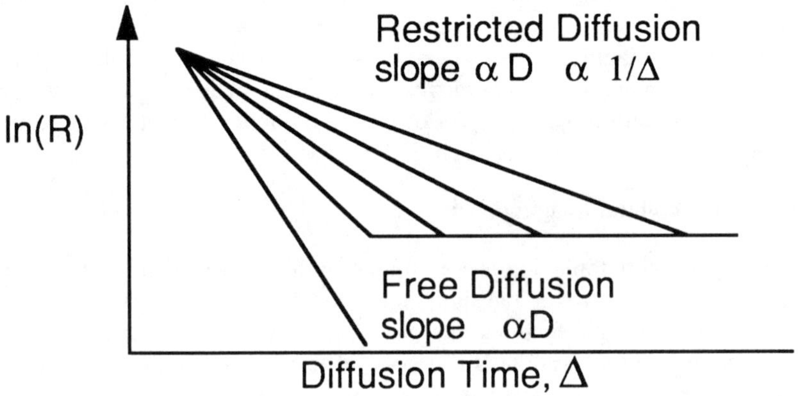

Figure 1.8. Decay of spin echo intensity as a function of diffusion time for a pulsed field gradient NMR experiment.

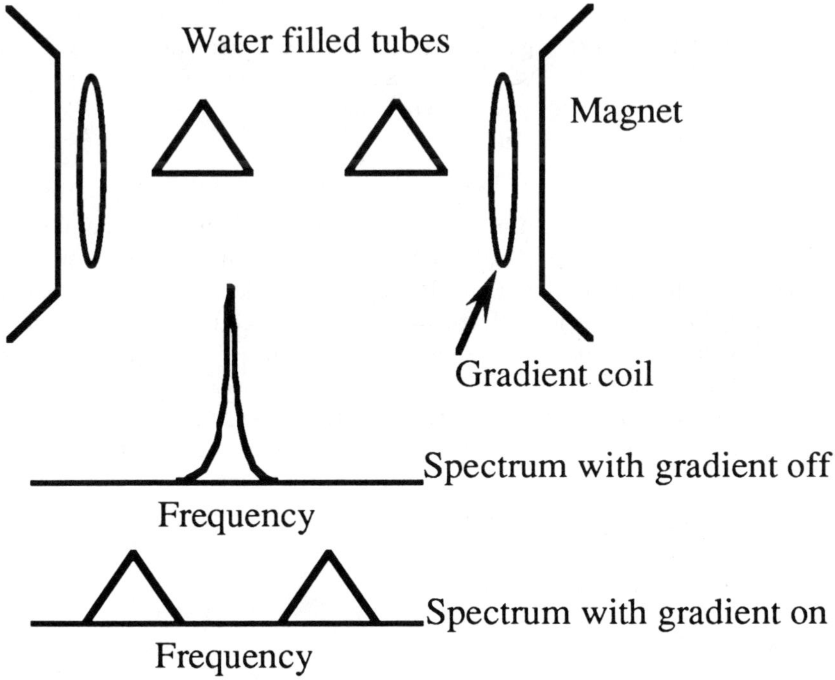

Figure 1.9. Influence of a linear magnetic field gradient on the NMR signal from two identical samples separated by a small distance inside the NMR probe.

This process of increasing the extent of the image can be continued to generate spatial information in two and even three dimensions; a two-dimensional image of an apple is shown in Figure 1.10. Different types of imaging techniques include density imaging, property-weighted imaging, chemical-shift imaging, q-space imaging, p-space imaging, diffusion-weighted imaging, velocity-weighted imaging, and microscopy. Examples of the use of these different MRI techniques will be given in Chapters 3 through 6.

Property-weighted Imaging

Property-weighted imaging is a term used in this book to define a two-dimensional MRI spectrum where the signal intensity characterizes a particular feature of the sample. Specific features that can be displayed as variations in intensity include component saturation, diffusion coefficient, temperature, and velocity. Analysis of property-weighted images provides information on heat transfer, mass transfer, fluid rheology, structure, and stability of a food system.

Chemical Shift Imaging

A chemical-shift image is a multi-dimensional data set consisting of a spatially resolved high-resolution NMR spectrum. In the simplest form, this is a two-dimensional data set with spatial position along one axis and chemical shift information along the other axis. This is a useful procedure for determining the distribution of oil and water in cheese or salad dressings.

Microscopy

NMR microscopy refers to an NMR image with volume elements (voxels) with dimensions $\leq (100\ \mu m)^3$ (Callaghan 1991). The fundamentals of image formation and the description of nuclear spin interactions remain the same as for standard MRI. The major differences are the increased influence on the NMR signal of molecular diffusion, spin-spin relaxation, magnetic susceptibility, and a reduced signal-to-noise ratio. NMR microscopy will be useful in understanding the development of stress cracks in grains, in determining the structure of foods on a length scale previously difficult to probe, and in examining interfaces.

Applications and Impact of MRI on Food Research

Food Stability and Structure

Foams

Both the dynamics and the structure of foams are easily studied using MRI. The gas or liquid phase volume fraction can be measured as a function of height

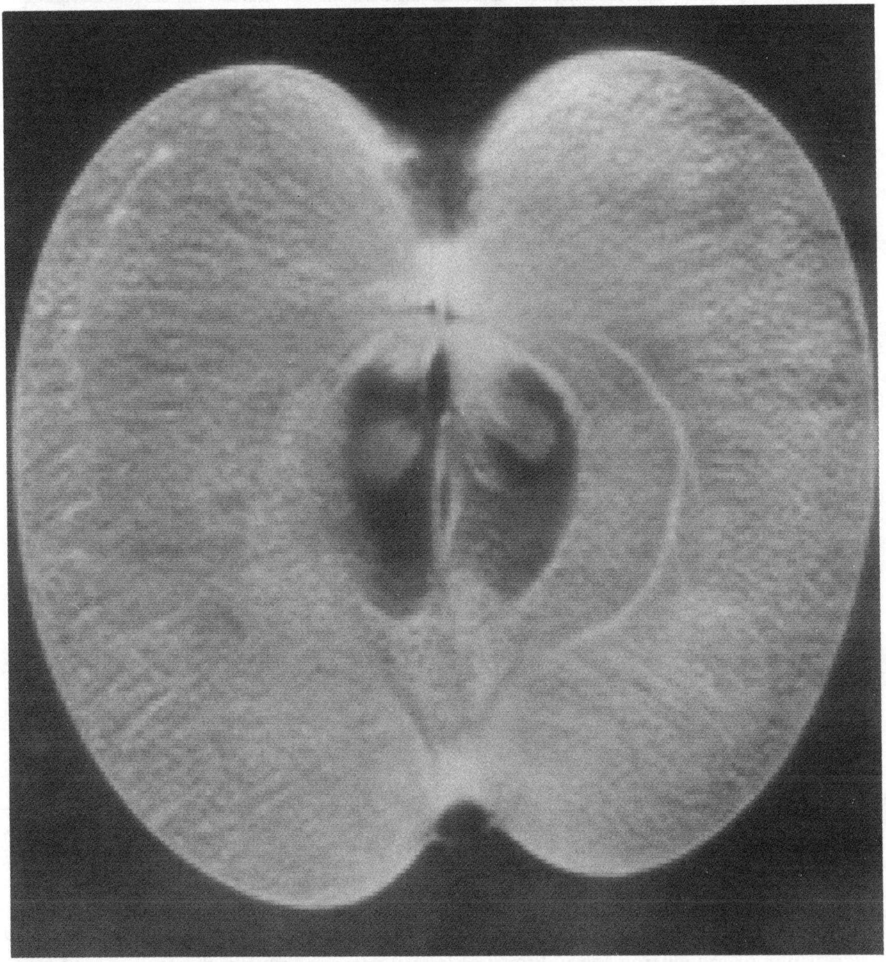

Figure 1.10. Proton density magnetic resonance image of an apple.

and time as shown in Figure 1.11. Egg white foam has been used as a model of a stable foam for comparison of measured liquid density profiles to theoretical predictions (McCarthy & Heil 1990). The comparison demonstrated that a simple physical model of foam drainage did not even qualitatively predict increases in liquid density at the bottom of a draining foam. In most foams, both liquid drainage and bubble collapse contribute to destabilization. Liquid drainage is quantified by measuring the decrease in nuclei density as a function of height, while bubble collapse is partially quantified by measuring the decrease in foam column height (German & McCarthy 1989).

More extensive NMR experiments in the future may prove useful for quantify-

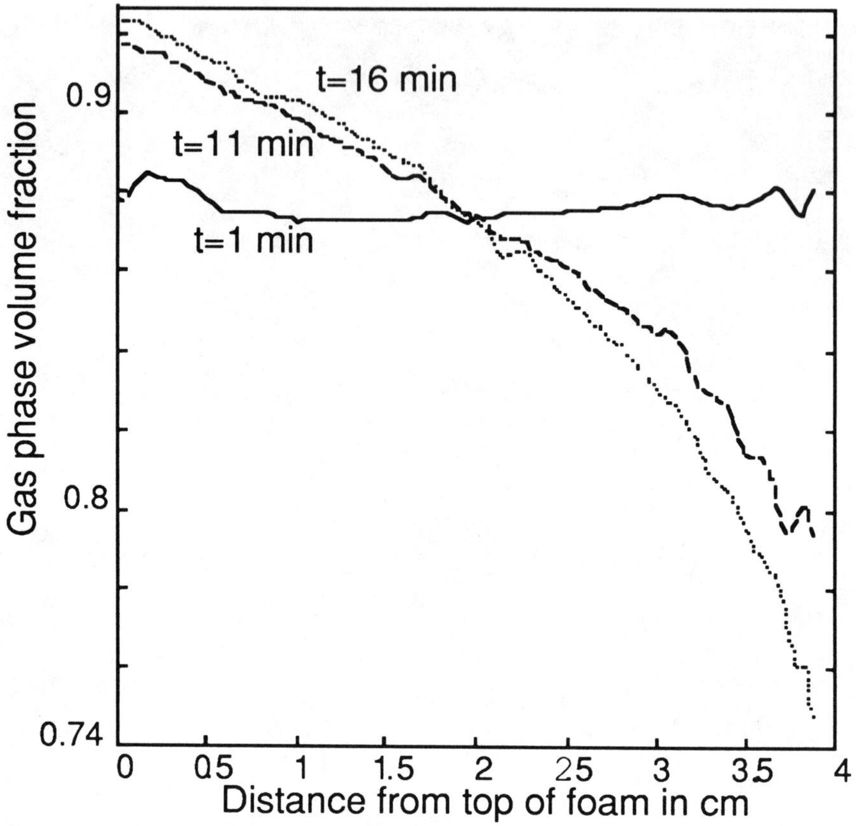

Figure 1.11. Gas phase volume fraction as a function of height in an egg white foam.

ing bubble size distribution by measuring the influence of magnetic susceptibility variations or measuring the velocity of liquid drainage within the foam. Additionally, coupling of MRI data with information from other experimental techniques (such as pressure and conductance measurements) should provide new information on the formation and destabilization of foams.

Emulsions

Measuring the droplet size distribution or concentration profiles in emulsions can be accomplished by using NMR techniques. Droplet size distributions can be quantified through application of PFGSE measurements of restricted diffusion (Lonnqvist, Kahn & Soderman 1991; Van Den Enden et al. 1990). The volume fractions of components as a function of height can be measured using a relaxation weighted image or a chemical shift image (Kauten, Maneval & McCarthy 1991).

The relaxation weighting technique is especially useful for rapidly destabilizing emulsions.

Characterization of emulsions can be improved by combining PFGSE and MRI pulse sequences in order to obtain droplet size distributions as a function of position and time. Combined with concentration profiles, this is a strong test of theoretical models as well as being an excellent tool for characterization of samples during stability tests. Combining the NMR droplet size distribution measurements with ultrasound measurements allows the relative influence of coalescence and flocculation to be determined (Stephanie Dungan, conversation with author 1992).

Gels

The morphology, molecular motion of solutes, state of water, and biopolymer concentration variations in gels have all been effectively studied using NMR techniques (Duce, Carpenter & Hall 1990a; Hills, Cano & Belton 1991). The extension of these studies to characterizing gel systems on a spatially resolved basis is just beginning. Spatial maps of gel structure based on variations in spin-spin relaxation times provide a means of measuring solute concentration variations in intact gels and composite foods (Duce, Carpenter & Hall 1990a).

The continued application of these recently developed imaging approaches should provide an improved understanding of the heterogeneity of gel structure and the formation of this structure. For example, the curd shrinkage and whey migration during cheese production can be quantified with a standard spin-warp imaging pulse sequence as shown in Figure 1.12. Coupling this with multiple 180° pulses and a water proton spin-spin relaxation theory (Hills, Takacs & Belton 1989a,b) may provide a better quantification of the kinetics of gel formation and the structural changes during formation.

Moisture Migration

Dehydration/Rehydration

Measuring moisture content and moisture movement was suggested by Mansfield and Morris (1982) as an application of MRI to food science. The initial studies of the drying of agricultural products (apples and corn) were published in the late 1980's (Perez, Kauten & McCarthy 1988; Song & Litchfield 1989). In extensions of these initial studies, the moisture profiles have been analyzed in terms of effective diffusivities (McCarthy, Perez & Özilgen 1991; Schrader & Litchfield 1992). In addition to dehydration, rehydration of potatoes and dry beans has been studied (Heil, McCarthy & Özilgen 1992; Ruan et al. 1991). The studies of food materials done so far have not provided any dramatic improvements in the understanding of mass transfer in food materials.

Improvements in understanding drying phenomena will probably best be

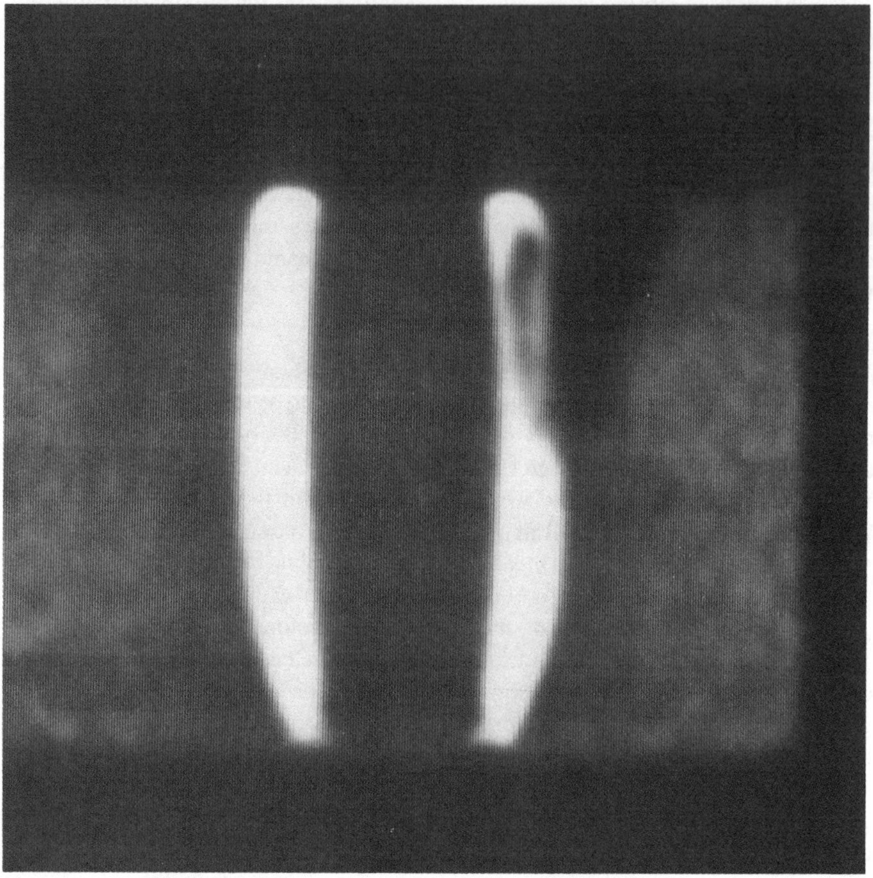

Figure 1.12. MRI of moisture migration after the cutting of a gel.

achieved by combining mathematical modeling of drying with measurements of the internal moisture profile and measurements of the state of water. An initial study combining this approach has indicated that the constant rate period of drying in porous media occurs because of the existence of films on the surface of the media and the first falling rate period can be well described with a model based on a surface with wet and dry regions (Maneval 1991).

Storage

The quality and consumer acceptance of many food products is in part determined by the amount of lipid and moisture migration that occurs during storage. Only demonstrations of the ability of MRI to quantify this process have been published to date (Duce, Carpenter & Hall 1990b; McCarthy & Kauten 1990).

Relaxation time weighted images are particularly useful for visualizing the movement of moisture. A relaxation time weighted image provides information primarily on the spatial distribution of one component in a complex mixture.

Future applications of MRI in studying moisture/lipid transport will probably be combined with the development of transport barrier films. These films are being developed to prevent or reduce moisture migration and the effectiveness of the film could be monitored *in situ* with MRI.

Rheology

MRI is becoming one of the premier experimental tools for studying the flow of fluids and suspensions. The applications are still in their early stages and have already yielded important information. With MRI, the velocity profiles within opaque fluids as well as the velocity profiles and particulate profiles in suspensions can be measured in tube flow (Altobelli, Givler & Fukushima 1991; Sinton & Chow 1991). These studies have shown that particle distributions can be nonuniform and recent work on simulated food suspension has quantified the influence of moderate particle loadings on fluid velocity profiles (K. McCarthy, personal communication). This information will be particularly important for improving models of heat transfer for aseptic processing. The flow of fluids in complex geometries such as between the screw and the barrel of an extruder have recently been demonstrated (McCarthy, Kauten & Agemura 1992). The flow of CMC solution in a single-screw extruder is shown in Figure 1.13.

Applications of MRI flow measurements will likely expand to include laminar to turbulent transitions, flow in twin-screw extruders, flow in dies, and flow in other complex geometries. Currently, the application of flow measurements is proceeding faster than the development of a precise mathematical method of analysis of the data and of procedures to convert velocity profiles into standard rheological information. The mathematical analysis of the pulse sequences and the conversion of MRI velocity information is critical to making advances in understanding the fluid dynamics occurring in food processing equipment.

Phase Changes

Freezing

MRI has been used to follow the movement of the ice interface in foods during freezing (McCarthy et al. 1991). This data is based on changes in signal intensity between unfrozen regions (high signal) and frozen regions (low signal) as shown in Figure 1.14. Comparison between estimates of the enthalpy of partially-frozen beef based on MRI data and measured values using a calorimeter have shown excellent agreement (M. McCarthy, unpublished results).

The agreement between MRI enthalpy estimates and actual values may allow for the development of an MRI-based sensor for control of industrial freezing

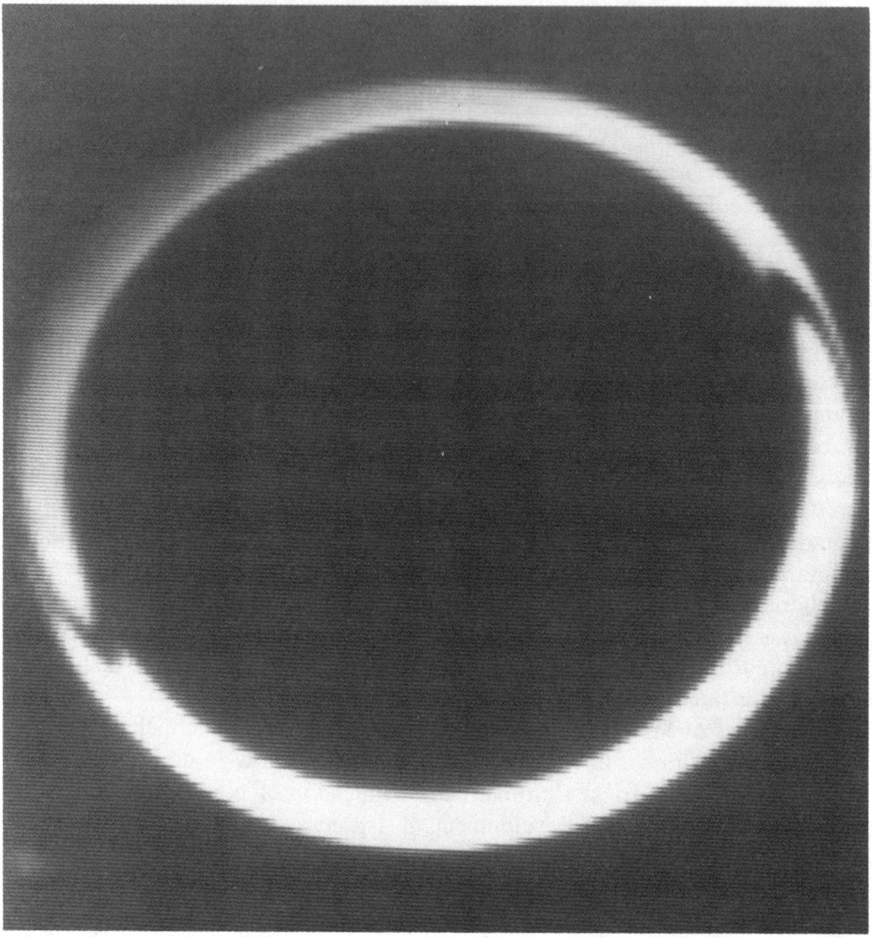

Figure 1.13. Velocity profile of CMC solution flowing between the screw and the barrel of a plastic single-screw extruder.

processes, as well as optimization of freezer design. Details of the structure of the ice interface are apparent in MRI data; however, this ice/liquid interface region has yet to be analyzed in detail. Analysis of this interface data may improve the physical description of freezing in tissues.

Lipid Crystallization

MRI has been used to study lipid crystallization in both model food systems and actual foods (Duce, Carpenter & Hall 1990b; Simoneau et al. 1991; Simoneau et al. 1993). These studies have demonstrated that MRI can be used to measure

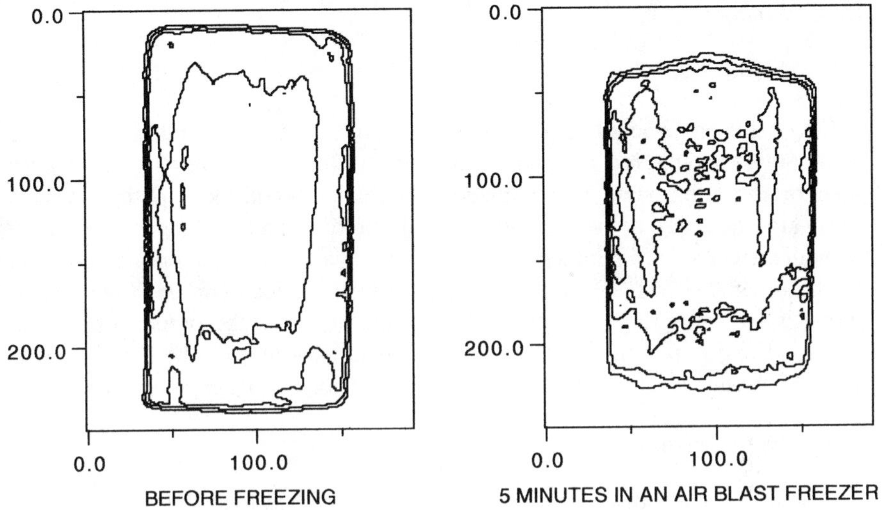

Figure 1.14. MRI of freezing process in a carrot.

the kinetics of crystallization, solid/liquid ratio, polymorphism, and fat structure. The NMR-based techniques complement existing experimental techniques such as DSC and X-ray diffraction. MRI is particularly effective in measuring the kinetics of fat crystallization in complex foods and in determining the influence of fat dispersion on crystallization (Özilgen et al. 1993).

The use of MRI techniques along with existing experimental approaches should provide important new information on the role of fat in product texture, structure, stability, and organoleptic properties. As in the control of freezing processes, MRI would be a useful process control monitor for lipid crystallization in complex foods.

Capabilities and Limitations of MRI

In this section the commonly achievable types of experiments and information available will be described. *Commonly achievable* means those that can be measured using a commercial research grade instrument without special programming. Common to all experiments is the fact that MRI is noninvasive and nondestructive. This allows for very efficient data gathering since several identical experiments stopped at different times to characterize transient conditions are unnecessary. Typical experiments measure a component density, component diffusivities, bulk flow of a fluid, mobility of a component, or provide a measure of the internal structure of a system.

Density Imaging

Temperature Range

MRI data can be acquired over almost all ranges of temperatures and pressures commonly encountered in food processing or storage. However, the physical state of the component to be imaged should be liquid-like. Without special hardware, gases are not sufficiently dense to produce an NMR signal. Similarly, without special experimental protocols and hardware, solid-like components cannot be imaged. Thus, while a strong signal from a bread can be obtained, this signal is from the mobile water and lipid and not from the other components. In a food that is frozen, a strong, liquid-like signal can often be observed even at very low temperatures, indicating that not all of the water phase is ice.

Moisture Content Range

Systems of glass beads and water have been studied over the range of 0.1% to 100% moisture saturation (Maneval 1991). The commonly encountered range of moistures in food can be easily studied. Difficulties in reaching fine spatial resolution ($<100\ \mu m$ in-plane) can occur in lower moisture systems. This limitation in spatial resolution is a result of the sample-spectrometer interactions and will be discussed in detail in Chapter 2.

Diffusion/Flow Imaging

Diffusivity Range

Diffusivities of ^1H containing molecules can be measured down to about 10^{-14} $m^2\ s^{-1}$ (Callaghan 1991). The accuracy of the measurement on a well-calibrated spectrometer should be on the order of 0.1% with the sample being a homogeneous liquid (Callaghan 1991). Accuracy will be decreased in more complex systems.

Velocity Range

A wide range of velocity measurements have been reported, ranging from 5m/s (Kuethe 1989) to 10^{-3} cm/sec (Holtz, Muller & Wachter 1986). The range of velocities available on a spectrometer will depend upon the gradient strength, size of the magnet's homogeneous field region, and the relaxation properties of the material. The range of flow rates easily measured by the author on a standard imaging spectrometer without shielded gradients is 10^{-2} m/s to 0.8 m/s.

Temperature Imaging

The mapping of temperature using MRI has been performed using variations in spin-lattice relaxation and diffusion coefficients (Le Bihan, Delannoy & Levin

1989). Spin-lattice relaxation maps of temperature have about a 2°C accuracy (Parker et al. 1983) and diffusivity maps provide about 1°C accuracy (Le Bihan, Delannoy & Levin 1989). The samples studied so far include gels, fluids, and muscle. The component to be studied needs to be in a liquid-like state. Since the approach based on the variation of the diffusion coefficient with temperature has better accuracy, this is the method of choice. The Stokes-Einstein relationship between diffusivity and liquid viscosity is used to develop an equation relating diffusivity to temperature. Many assumptions are involved in developing the relationship and thus estimating the range of temperatures that can be studied is not simple. It appears that for model food gels, the range of temperatures that currently can be studied are from approximately −5°C to 70°C. This is an area where rapid development should occur and the range should be expanded soon.

Structural Imaging

The structure that is displayed in MRI data is digital in nature. Each voxel is an integrated signal that can be influenced by component density, component relaxation times, motion, and experimental parameters in the pulse sequence. Therefore, the structure or contrast displayed in an image can be modified in a large number of ways and the interpretation of the structure observed needs to include the manner in which the structure or contrast is achieved.

Voids

Bubbles, voids, solids, and air pockets do not provide sufficient NMR signals to be recorded in typical MRI experiments. The effect on the image is then to provide a region with no signal or reduced signal intensity. A reduced signal results when a bubble is smaller than the voxel or is situated between two or more voxels, as shown in Figure 1.15.

The influence of voids on signal intensity can be used to measure total void volume and characteristics of the voids. These characteristics include size distribution and spatial distribution.

Water and/or Lipid

In most food systems, the component density and/or the spatial distribution can be measured with precision. In foods that have water or lipid as the major component contributing to the NMR signal, the component density is often proportional to the signal. The constant of proportionality may be a function of relaxation rates; however, this can be corrected by the procedures described in Chapter 2.

If both lipid and water contribute significantly to the NMR signal, chemical shift imaging should be used to quantify component densities. However, this adds an additional dimension to the data set and significant time to the experiment.

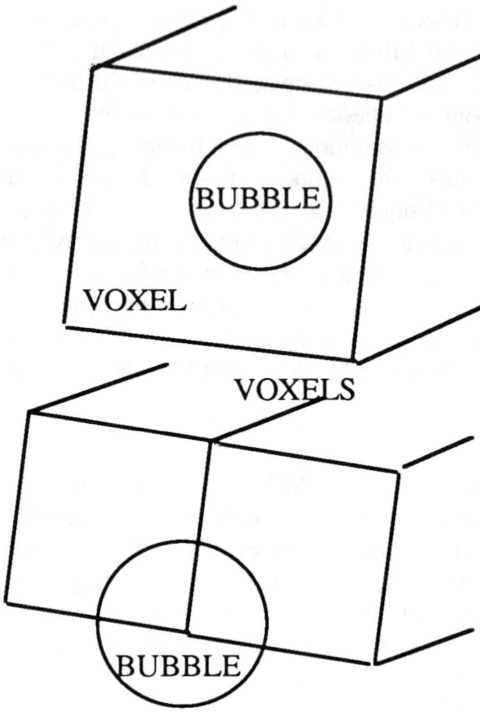

Figure 1.15. Relative positions of air bubbles with respect to voxels.

Most importantly, the density measured in NMR experiments is ^{1}H nuclei density per volume element. The conversion to weight per weight of dry solids is often difficult. Current MRI techniques do not allow for quantification of liquid-like and solid-like signals when both are present.

Spatial distribution of lipid and water can often be obtained using relaxation time weighted images. These are effective as long as either the spin-lattice or spin-spin relaxation times differ significantly for the two components. Shown in Figure 1.16 is the MRI image of an intact trout with the lipid signal intensity enhanced relative to the water signal intensity.

Chemical Shift Effect

The slightly different resonance absorption frequencies for different components can result in image artifacts which are manifest as spatial misregistrations. For example, if a one-dimensional frequency encoding of the signal is performed on a vial of oil and water with the phases separated, the expected result is a one-dimensional density profile of the vial. However, this profile is distorted as

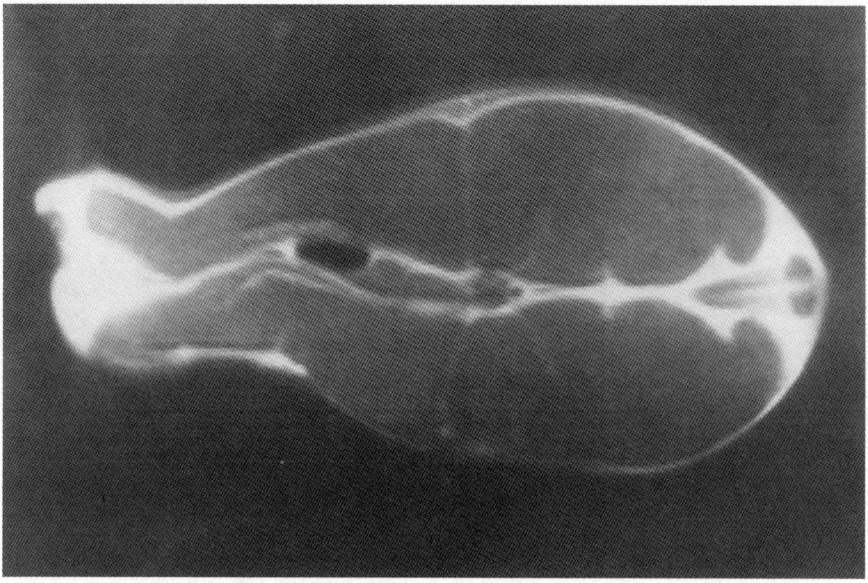

Figure 1.16. Fat-weighted MRI of the central region of an intact trout.

shown in Figure 1.17. The overlap arises from the small difference in absorption frequencies quantified by the chemical shift difference between oil and water. Thus, in two-dimensional MRI experiments, chemical shift artifacts are often apparent as thin bright lines. In many instances, this known characteristic can be used to locate oil-water interfaces.

Magnetic Susceptibility Effect

The total magnetic field in a sample placed within a magnet is proportional to the strength of the applied field plus the amount of magnetization within the sample induced by the applied external field. The magnitude of the magnetization is given by the product of the magnetic susceptibility and the external magnetic field strength. The total magnetic field experienced by nuclei within a sample is then the sum of the external field and the internal field generated by the material. Different materials have different magnetic susceptibilities and this results in differences in the local magnetic field within heterogeneous materials like foams. The artifacts generated in images by these extra magnetic field gradients are either decreases in signal or bright spots. The decrease in signal occurs because the magnetic susceptibility differences tend to increase the effective spin-spin rate and hence decrease the intensity of the NMR signal. As in chemical shift effects, the bright spots or lines occur due to spatial misregistration.

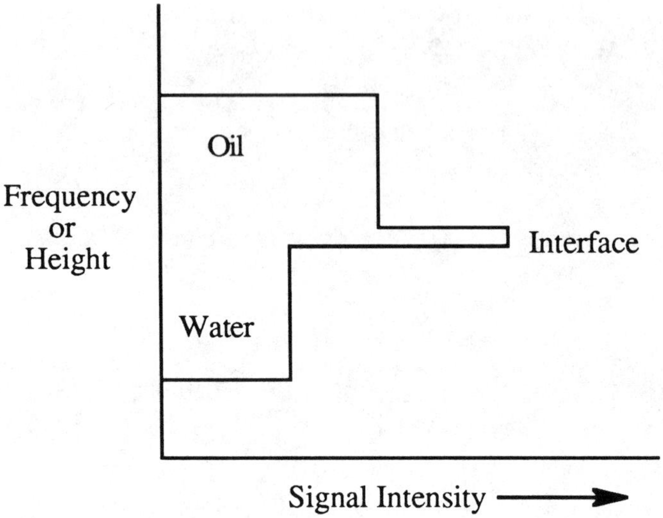

Figure 1.17. Ideal one-dimensional profile of oil on top of water.

Image Resolution

Spatial

In a two-dimensional image (Figure 1.12), there are three measurements that need to be specified in order to define voxel size. The voxel can be thought of as a cubic volume which is calculated by multiplying slice thickness (z direction) by length of voxel in the frequency encode direction (x direction) by phase encode direction (y direction). A typical voxel dimension is 2 mm by 0.2 mm by 0.2 mm. With normal strength gradients, the smallest cubic voxel would have an edge length of 0.2 mm. For microscopy applications, the voxel size is much smaller, often on the order of 10–20 μm (Callaghan 1991). The ultimate resolution obtainable using MRI microscopy techniques should be on the order of 2 μm (Callaghan 1991); however, this is dependent on the sample characteristics and on the spectrometer.

Temporal

The speed of acquiring MRI data varies significantly depending on the type of magnetic field gradient coils available and on the sample to be studied (Mansfield & Morris 1982). Magnetic field gradients can be either shielded or unshielded. Shielded gradients can be turned off and on more rapidly and induce fewer artifacts in the data than unshielded gradients. A detailed description of shielded gradients is given in Chapter 3. For MRI spectrometers without shielded gradients, rapid two-dimensional images can be acquired in a few seconds. If a spectrometer has shielded gradients, similar information can be acquired in approximately 50 ms using echo-planar techniques. For one-dimensional MRI data, either system can acquire the information in approximately 10 ms. Generally, if a sample has a short spin-spin relaxation time, echo-planar techniques are not effective in acquiring adequate signal. However, advances in application of echo-planar techniques have shown that good images of species with short spin-spin relaxation times is possible (Guilfoyle, Mansfield & Packer 1992).

References

Abragam, A. 1961. *Principles of nuclear magnetism.* New York: Oxford University Press.

Altobelli, S. A., Givler, R. C., & Fukushima, E. 1991. Velocity and concentration measurements of suspensions by nuclear magnetic resonance imaging. *J. of Rheology* **35**: 721–734.

Barrall, G. A., Frydman, L., & Chingas, G. C. 1992. NMR diffraction and spatial statistics of stationary systems. *Science* **255**: 714–717.

Bloch, F. 1946. Nuclear induction. *Physical Review* **70**: 460–474.

Callaghan, P. T. 1991. *Principles of nuclear magnetic resonance microscopy.* New York: Oxford University Press.

Duce, S. L., Carpenter, T. A., & Hall, L. D. 1990a. Use of n.m.r. imaging to map the spatial distrubution [*sic*] of structure in polysaccharide gels. *Carbohydrate Research* C1-C4.

Duce, S. L., Carpenter, T. A., & Hall, L. D. 1990b. Nuclear magnetic resonance imaging of chocolate confectionery and the spatial detection of polymorphic states of cocoa butter in chocolate. *Lebensmittel-Wissenschaft und-Technologie* **23**: 565–569.

Ernst, R. R., Bodenhausen, G., & Wokaun, A. 1987. *Principles of nuclear magnetic resonance in one and two dimensions.* Oxford: Clarendon Press.

Gadian, D. G. 1982. *Nuclear magnetic resonance and its applications to living systems.* New York: Oxford University Press.

German, J. B., & McCarthy, M. J. 1989. Stability of aqueous foams: Analysis using magnetic resonance imaging. *J. of Agricultural and Food Chemistry* **37**: 1321–1324.

Guilfoyle, D. N., Mansfield, P., & Packer, K. J. 1992. Fluid flow measurement in porous media by echo-planar imaging. *J. of Magnetic Resonance* **97**: 342–358.

Heil, J. R., McCarthy, M. J., & Özilgen, M. 1992. Magnetic resonance imaging and modeling of water up-take into dry beans. *Lebensm.-Wiss. u.-Technol.* **25**: 280–285.

Hills, B. P., Cano, C., & Belton, P. S. 1991. Proton NMR relaxation studies of aqueous polysaccharide systems. *Macromolecules* **24**: 2944–2950.

Hills, B. P., Takacs, S. F., & Belton, P. S. 1989. The effects of proteins on the proton N.M.R. transverse relaxation times of water I. Native bovine serum albumin. *Molecular Physics* **67**: 903–918.

Hills, B. P., Takacs, S. F., & Belton, P. S. 1989. The effects of proteins on the proton N.M.R. transverse relaxation time of water II. Protein aggregation. *Molecular Physics* **67**: 919–937.

Holtz, M., Muller, C., & Wachter, A. M. 1986. Modification of the pulsed magnetic field gradient method for the determination of low velocities by NMR. *J. of Magnetic Reson.* **69**: 108–115.

Kauten, R. J., Maneval, J. E., & McCarthy, M. J. 1991. Fast determination of spatially localized volume fractions in emulsions. *J. of Food Science* **56**: 799–801, 847.

Kuethe, D. O. 1989. Measuring distributions of eddy diffusivity with magnetic resonance imaging. Seventh Symposium on Turbulent Shear Flows. Stanford University, Palo Alto, CA.

Lauterbur, P. C. 1973. Image formation by induced local interactions: Examples employing nuclear magnetic resonance. *Nature* **242**: 190–191.

Le Bihan, D., Delannoy, J., & Levin, R. L. 1989. Temperature mapping with MR imaging of molecular diffusion: Application to hyperthermia. *Radiology* **171**: 853–857.

Lonnqvist, I., Kahn, A., & Soderman, O. 1991. Characterization of emulsions by NMR methods. *J. of Colloid and Interface Science* **144**: 401–411.

Maneval, J. E. 1991. Ph.D. University of California, Davis.

Maneval, J. E., Powell, R. L., McCarthy, M. J., & McCarthy, K. L. 1992. Magnetic resonance imaging of multiphase systems. In *Particulate Two-Phase Flow*, edited by M. Roco, 127–140. Boston: Butterworth-Heinenann.

Mansfield, P., & Grannell, P. K. 1973. NMR 'diffraction' in solids? *J. of Physics C: Solid State Physics* **6**: L422-L426.

Mansfield, P., & Morris, P. G. 1982. *NMR imaging in biomedicine*. New York: Academic Press.

McCarthy, K. L., & Heil, J. R. 1990. Internal liquid flow during foam drainage: comparison of theory and experiment. In *Food Emulsion and Foams: Theory and Practice*, edited by P. J. Wan, J. L. Cavallo, F. Z. Saleeb, & M. J. McCarthy, 71–75. New York: American Institute of Chemical Engineers.

McCarthy, K. L., Kauten, R., & Agemura, C. 1992. Application of NMR imaging to the study of velocity profiles during extrusion processing. *Trends in Food Science and Technolgy* **3**: 215–219.

McCarthy, M. J., Charoenrein, S., German, J. B., McCarthy, K. L., & Reid, D. S. 1991. Phase volume measurements using magnetic resonance imaging. In *Water Relationships in Foods: Advances in the 1980s and Trends for the 1990s*, edited by H. Levine & L. Slade, 615–626. New York: Plenum Press.

McCarthy, M. J., & Kauten, R. J. 1990. Magnetic resonance imaging applications in food research. *Trends in Food Science and Technology* **1**: 134–139.

McCarthy, M. J., Perez, E., & Özilgen, M. 1991. Model for transient moisture profiles of a drying apple slab using the data obtained with magnetic resonance imaging. *Biotechnology Progress* **7**: 540–543.

Morris, P. G. 1986. *Nuclear Magnetic Resonance Imaging in Medicine and Biology*. New York: Oxford University Press.

Özilgen, S., Simoneau, C., German, J. B., McCarthy, M. J., & Reid, D. S. 1993. Crystallization kinetics of emulsified triglycerides. *J. of the Sci. of Food and Ag.* **61**: 101–108.

Parker, D. L., Smith, V., Sheldon, P., Crooks, L. E., & Fussel, L. 1983. Temperature distribution measurements in two-dimensional NMR imaging. *Med. Phys.* **10**: 321–325.

Perez, E., Kauten, R., & McCarthy, M. J. 1988. Noninvasive measurement of moisture profiles during the drying of an apple. Sixth Inter. Drying Symp. Versailles, France.

Ruan, R., Schmidt, S. J., Schmidt, A. R., & Litchfield, J. B. 1991. Nondestructive measurement of transient moisture profiles and the moisture diffusion coefficient in a potato during drying and absorption by NMR imaging. *J. of Food Process Engineering* **14**: 297–313.

Schmidt, S. J. 1991. Determination of moisture content by pulsed nuclear magnetic resonance spectroscopy. In *Water Relationships in Foods: Advances in the 1980s and Trends for the 1990s*, edited by H. Levine, & L. Slade, 599–613. New York: Plenum Press.

Schmidt, S. J., & Lai, H. 1991. Use of NMR and MRI to study water relations in foods. In *Water Relationships in Foods: Advances in the 1980s and Trends for the 1990s*, edited by H. Levine, & L. Slade, 405–452. New York: Plenum Press.

Schrader, G. W., & Litchfield, J. B. 1992. Moisture profiles in a model food gel during drying measurement using magnetic resonance imaging and evaluation of the Fickian odel. *Drying Technology* **10**: 295–332.

Simoneau, C., McCarthy, M. J., Kauten, R. J., & German, J. B. 1991. Crystallization dynamics in model emulsions from magnetic resonance imaging. *J. of the American Oil Chemists' Society* **68**: 481–487.

Simoneau, C., McCarthy, M. J., Reid, D. S., & German, J. B. 1993. Influence of triglyceride composition on crystallization kinetics of model emulsions. *J. of Food Engi.* **19**: 365–387.

Sinton, S. W., & Chow, A. W. 1991. NMR flow imaging of fluids and solid suspensions in Poiseuille flow. *J. of Rheology* **35**: 735–772.

Song, H., & Litchfield, J. B. 1989. Nondestructive measurement of transient, 3-D moisture transfer in corn during drying using NMR imaging. American Society of Agricultural Engineers. New Orleans, Louisiana.

Van Den Enden, J. C., Waddington, D., Van Aalst, H., Van Kralingen, C. G., & Packer, K. J. 1990. Rapid determination of water droplet size distribution by PFG-NMR. *J. of Colloid and Interface Science* **140**: 105–113.

2

Fundamental Principles of MRI

Quantum Mechanical Description of NMR

Accurate descriptions of the state of microscopic particles such as electrons, atoms, or nuclei generally require the use of quantum mechanics. For NMR experiments, the interaction of the nuclear magnetic moments with an applied internal field is used to examine the chemical environment within the sample. Magnetic moments arise from orbital angular momentum and spin angular momentum of a changed particle.

For a nuclear spin 1/2 system in an external magnetic field, the magnetic moments can be aligned with the external field or against the external field; this is shown in Figure 2.1 as different energy levels and is referred to as the Zeeman effect. The difference in the energy between the two levels is directly proportional to the applied external magnetic field strength. In an NMR experiment, transitions are induced between the two energy levels to displace the system from equilibrium. This displacement from equilibrium and the return to equilibrium is expressed mathematically using the Schrödinger equation and quantum mechanical operators. The quantum mechanical operators are called Hamiltonians and they are mathematical descriptions of the interactions between the nuclear spins and the surrounding lattice. The Hamiltonians for NMR can be divided into external and internal. External Hamiltonians include the effect of the external magnetic field, the linear magnetic field gradients, and RF pulses. Internal Hamiltonians describe interactions between the nuclear spins and magnetic fields within the sample; examples are chemical shift, spin-lattice interactions, and spin-spin couplings. The objective in every NMR experiment is to use the external Hamiltonians to measure the influence of one or more internal interactions. A simpler mathematical model for the interaction of nuclear magnetic moments with external magnetic fields is given by the Bloch model. For the majority of NMR imaging

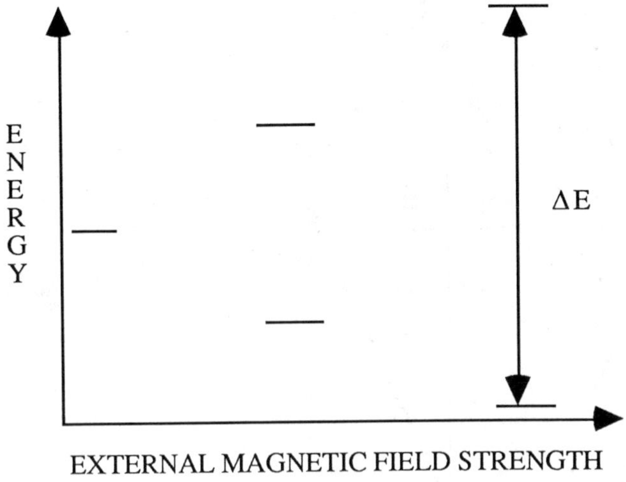

Figure 2.1. Energy levels in a spin 1/2 system.

studies, the interactions of spin 1/2 nuclei such as ^1H are adequately described by the Bloch model.

Bloch Model of NMR

Characteristics of Physical System for Which the Bloch Model is Correct

In NMR imaging, the nuclei within the samples being studied usually have liquid-like behavior. Thus, the nuclear magnetic moments (or spins) are noninteracting or only weakly interacting and the Bloch equation is used to describe the time evolution of the system (Bloch 1946). The Bloch equation was initially postulated to describe the behavior of an ensemble of spin 1/2 nuclei under the influence of a magnetic field:

$$\frac{d\mathbf{M}}{dt} = \gamma \mathbf{M} \times \mathbf{B} \qquad [2.1]$$

where γ is the gyromagnetic ratio, $\mathbf{B}$ is the external magnetic field, and $\mathbf{M}$ is the vector sum of the individual nuclear magnetic moments $\mathbf{I}_j$.

$$\mathbf{M} = \Sigma \mathbf{I}_j \qquad [2.2]$$

when $\mathbf{B} = B_o\mathbf{k}$; this is a coupled set of ordinary differential equations for $M_x\mathbf{i}$ and $M_y\mathbf{j}$. The solution of these equations is a precessional motion of the $\mathbf{M}$ about the direction of $\mathbf{B}$ as shown in Figure 2.2. The frequency of precession is given by the Larmor equation:

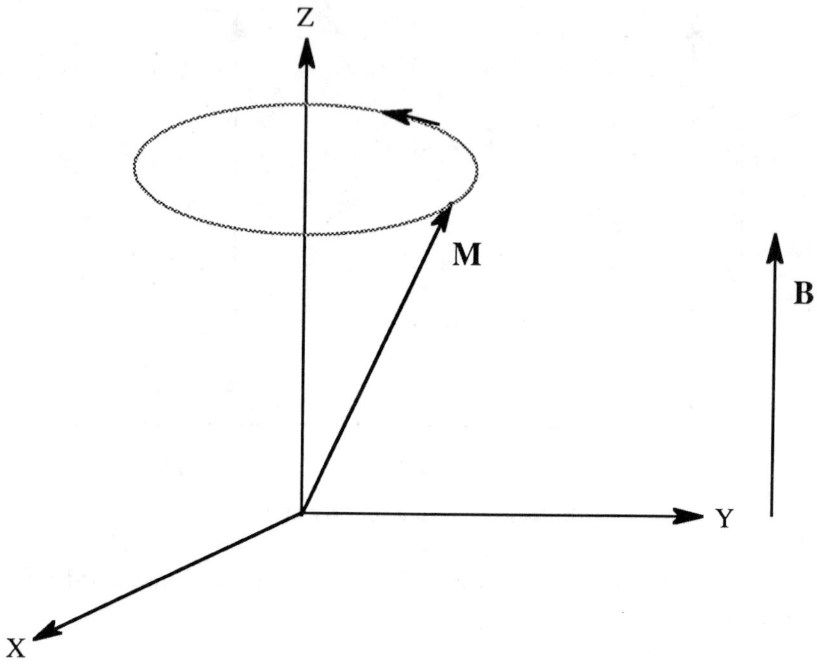

Figure 2.2. Precessional motion of the net macroscopic magnetic moment.

$$\omega_o = \gamma B_o \qquad [2.3]$$

(Clockwise rotations imply a positive ω_o.)

Relaxation Effects

Bloch originally observed that when the net magnetization was displaced from equilibrium, the system returned to its original state by following an exponential decay. This exponential response was observed for the decay of magnetization in the X-Y plane and for the return of magnetization along the Z-axis. Bloch then added these terms into the equation of motion for the nuclear spins (Bloch 1946):

$$\frac{d\mathbf{M}}{dt} = \gamma \mathbf{M} \times \mathbf{B} - \frac{M_x}{T_2}\mathbf{i} - \frac{M_y}{T_2}\mathbf{j} + \frac{(M_0 - M_z)}{T_1}\mathbf{k} \qquad [2.4]$$

where T_2 is the spin-spin relaxation time and T_1 is the spin-lattice relaxation time. The spin-spin relaxation time characterizes the entropic processes occurring and the spin-lattice relaxation time characterizes the enthalpic processes.

Analysis of an NMR experiment usually proceeds by transforming the Bloch equations into a rotating reference frame. The frame is chosen to rotate at the Larmor frequency and the Bloch equation then becomes:

$$\left.\frac{d\mathbf{M}}{dt}\right)_{rot} = \left.\frac{d\mathbf{M}}{dt}\right)_{lab} + \omega \times \mathbf{M} = \gamma\mathbf{M} \times \mathbf{B}_{eff} \qquad [2.5]$$

where $\mathbf{B}_{eff} = \mathbf{B} + (\omega_r/r)\mathbf{k}$. If $\omega_r = -\omega_o$, then

$$\mathbf{B}_{eff} = \mathbf{B}_1\mathbf{i} + \Delta B_0\mathbf{k} \qquad [2.6]$$

where ΔB_0 includes any variations in the local magnetic field such as chemical shift, magnetic susceptibility, and field gradients. $\mathbf{B}_1$ represents the RF field applied to displace the system from equilibrium and manipulate the spin system.

Pulse Sequences

A pulse sequence describes the time ordering of events in an NMR experiment. Every NMR experiment can be described and analyzed using a pulse sequence diagram which is a graphical representation of the time order of the application of RF and field gradient pulses and the acquisition of data. Common pulse sequences are described below.

One-Pulse

The simplest of NMR experiments is the one-pulse experiment. In a one-pulse experiment, a short RF pulse is applied to displace the nuclear spin system from equilibrium. The angle of rotation is generally 90° since this provides the largest signal. After the RF pulse, the data acquisition is turned on and the FID acquired. The pulse sequence timing diagram for the one-pulse experiment is shown in Figure 2.3.

The solution to the Bloch equation for the one-pulse experiment is:

$$\begin{aligned} M_x &= M_0 e^{-t/T_2} \cos\Delta\omega t \\ M_y &= M_0 e^{-t/T_2} \sin\Delta\omega t \\ M_z &= M_0(1 - e^{-t/T_1}) \end{aligned} \qquad [2.7a–c]$$

where, $\Delta\omega = \omega_0 - \omega$. The NMR spectrum is usually calculated by a Fourier transform of the transverse components:

$$F(\omega) = \rho \int_{-\infty}^{+\infty} e^{-i\omega t} e^{-t/T_2} (\cos\Delta\omega t + i\sin\Delta\omega t) dt \qquad [2.8]$$

Assuming that the receiver phase offset = 0, integration yields a complex Lorentzian lineshape:

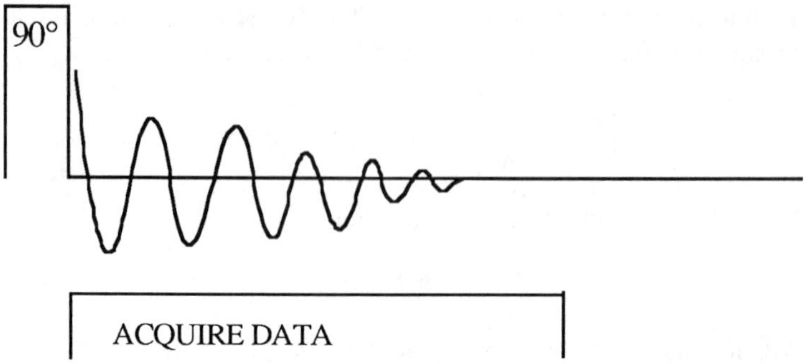

Figure 2.3. Pulse sequence timing diagram for a one-pulse experiment.

$$\mathrm{Re} = \frac{T_2}{1+(\omega-\Delta\omega)^2 T_2^2} \qquad [2.9]$$

$$\mathrm{Im} = \frac{-(\omega-\Delta\omega)T_2^2}{1+(\omega-\Delta\omega)^2 T_2^2}$$

The T_2 of the sample governs the linewidth as shown in the above equation. The smaller the value of T_2, the broader the line. This has an influence in MRI in terms of limiting the spatial resolution in the frequency encode direction. Often highly viscous or low moisture foods have broad NMR lines and thus the spatial resolution is limited in the frequency encode direction.

Spin Echo

Spin echoes arise in multiple pulse experiments as a result of the physics of the nuclear magnetic spin system. Figure 2.4 illustrates the pulse sequence diagram for the basic Hahn spin echo experiment. The basic pulse sequence consists of a 90° X pulse which rotates the net macroscopic magnetic moment about the X axis by 90°. The resulting magnetic moment and signal are along the positive Y axis. Next, the individual magnetic moments begin to dephase or lose phase coherence. This loss in phase coherence results from magnet field nonhomogeneities, chemical shift effects, magnetic susceptibility variations, spin-spin relaxation, and other effects which result in slightly different local magnetic fields within the sample. The variations in the local magnetic field give rise to differences in the precessional frequencies of the individual magnetic moments and the resulting vector sum (net macroscopic magnetic moment) decreases in time. The maximum magnitude of the spin echo is given by:

$$M(TE) = M_0 \exp\left\{\left[-TE/T_2\right] - 2/3\gamma^2 G^2 D (TE/2)^3\right\} \qquad [2.10]$$

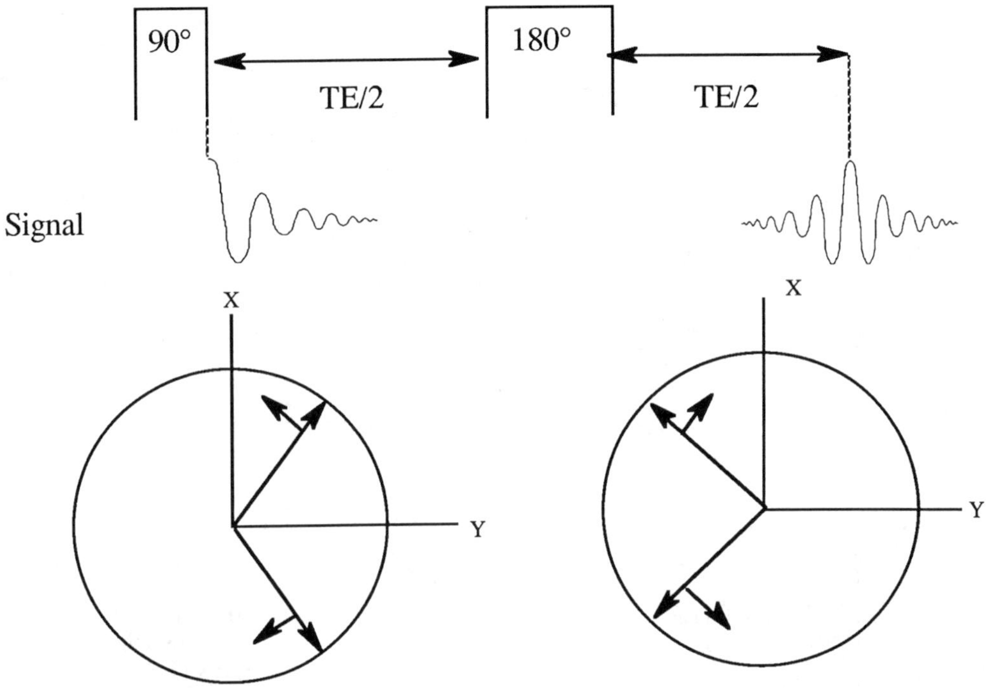

Figure 2.4. Pulse sequence timing diagram and motion of individual nuclear magnetic moments for a Hahn spin echo experiment.

where TE is the time from the center of the initial RF pulse to the echo center, G is magnetic field gradient strength, and D is the self-diffusion coefficient (Fukushima & Roeder 1981). For short values of TE, the effect of diffusion is small; however, as TE becomes large, the diffusion attenuation can become quite large. For more accurate measurements of T_2, a multiple pulse experiment using a train of equally spaced 180° pulses is recommended. This essentially eliminates the influence of diffusion on the signal attenuation (Carr & Purcell 1954). Care must be taken in interpreting the relaxation times from these multiple experiments because the spin-spin relaxation time for hydrogen can depend upon pulse spacing (Belton & Hills 1987). This results from diffusion and exchange of hydrogen between water and macromolecules. The variation of the spin-spin relaxation time with pulse spacing may provide a method for imaging the state of water in foods in terms of the actual dynamics of the interaction between water and macromolecules. Spin echoes are also important because the concept of phase is easily described. The phase of the NMR signal is the initial angle of the magnetization vector with respect to the Y axis (for the description in this book). This is shown in Figure 2.5. For the spin echo experiment, the phase of a spin can be followed using a spin phase map. Figure 2.6 is a plot of ϕ, the phase of

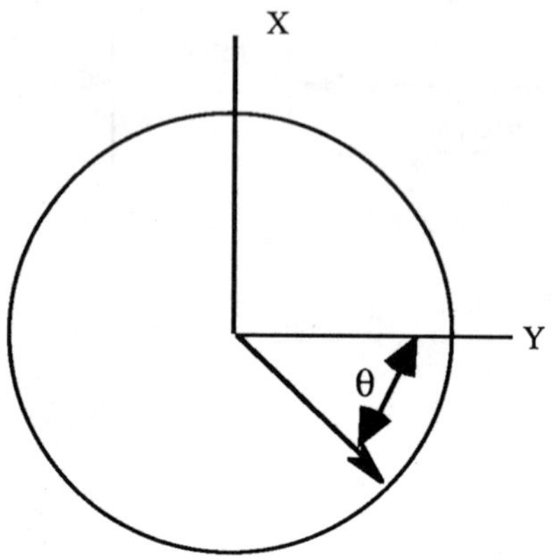

Figure 2.5. The phase of the NMR signal is the angle θ.

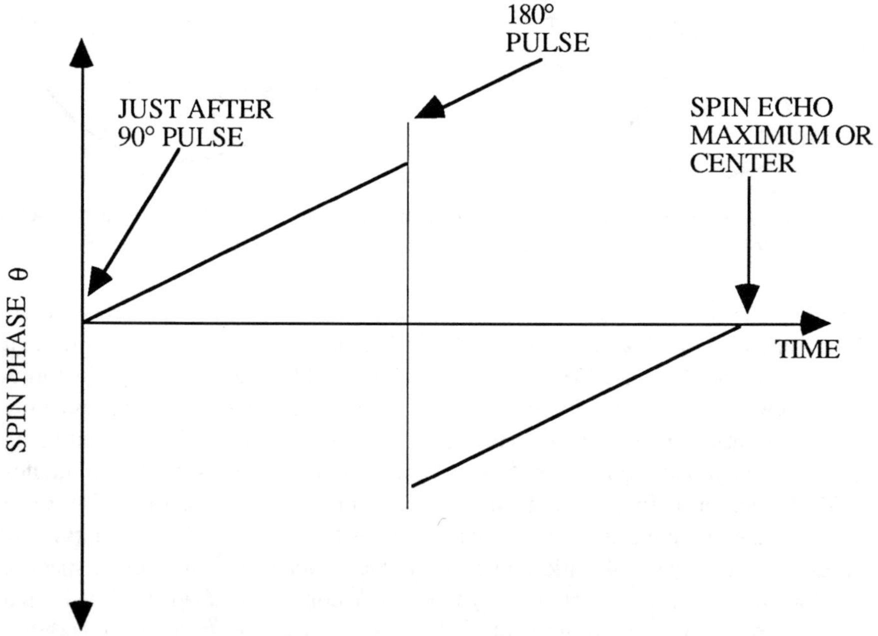

Figure 2.6. Spin phase plot for a Hahn spin echo pulse sequence.

the spin as a function of time. If the initial spin is aligned with the Y axis, the beginning value is zero. If the spin's precessional frequency differs from the rotational frequency of the rotating frame, the spin magnetization vector moves with respect to the Y axis. If the rotation is clockwise, the phase is a positive value and increases linearly with time (ignoring all other effects such as diffusion and/or flow which would change the precessional frequency). The 180° pulse inverts the sign of the phase. At this time the phase starts to decrease and reaches zero for the spin echo maximum.

Stimulated Echo

Echoes can also be formed using only 90° pulses. Figure 2.7 is the pulse sequence diagram for a stimulated echo (Hahn 1950) which is the first echo after the third 90° pulse. The other echoes are spin echoes and can be predicted by analysis of the pulse sequence.

The magnitude of the stimulated echo is:

$$M(\tau_2 + \tau_1) = \left(\frac{M_0}{2}\right) \exp(-2\tau_1/T_2) \exp(-(\tau_2 - \tau_1)/T_1) \qquad [2.11]$$

This is a useful pulse sequence for flow and diffusion imaging for materials with short T_2 relaxation times because the magnetization is stored along the Z axis and consequently decays as T_1 instead of as T_2.

Magnetic Resonance Imaging

In the process of acquiring the data to generate a typical NMR image, a pulse sequence can be divided into three stages:

1. Slice selection
2. Phase encoding
3. Frequency encoding

A linear magnetic field gradient is used to accomplish each stage of the experiment. The influence of the linear magnetic field gradient can be described by noting the change in the Larmor equation:

$$\omega_0 = \gamma B_0$$

If a linear field gradient is applied, the resonant frequency becomes a function of position:

$$\omega_0(\mathbf{r}) = \gamma B_0 + \gamma \mathbf{G}\cdot\mathbf{r} \qquad [2.12]$$

Since $|\mathbf{G}| << |B_0|$, only components of $\mathbf{G}$ parallel to B_0 are important for most imaging and microscopy experiments. If $\mathbf{G} = G_x\mathbf{i}$ then:

$$\Delta\omega = \gamma G_x \Delta x \qquad [2.13]$$

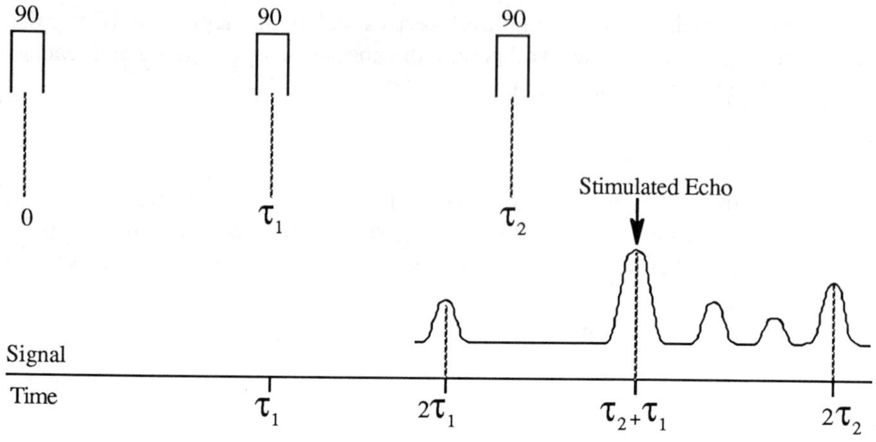

Figure 2.7. Pulse sequence timing diagram for a stimulated echo experiment.

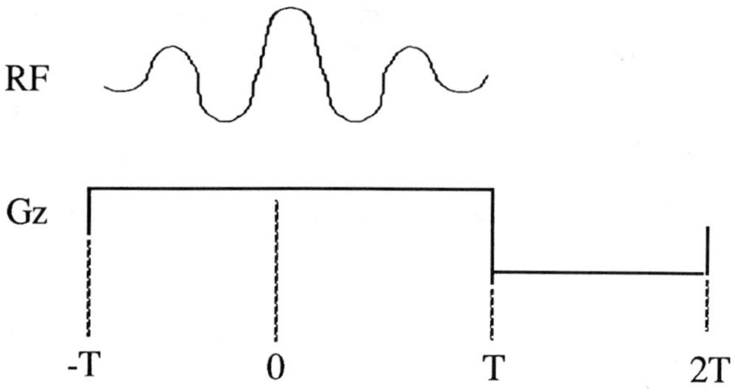

Figure 2.8. Components of slice selection, a selective pulse, and a linear field gradient.

This shows that spatial differences are proportional to differences in frequency. The stronger the gradient, the greater the range of frequencies over a finite sample size.

Slice Selection

The goal of slice selection is to define a plane of known thickness from the sample by use of a linear magnetic field gradient and a selective pulse; this is illustrated in Figure 2.8. A selective pulse is one which has a discrete band of frequencies. The gradient causes a large variation in the Larmor frequencies across the sample. The selective pulse normally has a narrower range of frequencies than that induced by a linear field gradient. Thus, the application of a narrow frequency range pulse results in displacing from equilibrium only spins in a narrow spatial range of the sample. The ideal selective pulse would result in a plane with parallel sides or with the following slice profile:

$$Sp(Z) = \begin{cases} 1 & |Z - Z_0| \leq L/2 \\ 0 & |Z - Z_0| > L/2 \end{cases} \quad [2.14]$$

where Sp is the fraction of nuclear spins excited at position Z, L is the slice thickness, and Z_0 is the center of the slice. This idealized slice geometry is generally not achieved. Usually some spins outside the plane are excited and spins within the plane are not uniformly exited. In most cases, the width of the slice is well defined and the out-of-plane excitations minor; an exception is 180° selective pulses. The RF pulse is shaped in order to produce a frequency profile as square as possible. A truncated sinc function or a sinc function multiplied by a Gaussian is normally used. For the sinc function, the bandwidth is determined by the pulse time t_p and is expressed as $\Delta\omega = 2\pi n/t_p$, with n being the number of cycles in the sinc function (Morris 1986). The degree of rotation is altered by changing the amplitude of the sinc function (amplification of the RF pulse).

After slice selection, only a single plane of spins is selected from a three-dimensional sample. The next procedure is to encode spatial information in the two dimensions orthogonal to the slice. This is accomplished by the application of a linear field gradient along these two directions for short periods of time.

Phase Encoding

Phase encoding is a process where the spatial distribution of the spin density is encoded in the phase of the NMR signal. For a spin echo-based Fourier imaging sequence, a gradient is applied for a short period of time, t_y. This gradient creates the following distribution of phase angles across the sample:

$$\begin{aligned} \phi(y) &= \gamma \Delta B t_y \\ \Delta B &= G_y y \\ \phi(y) &= \gamma G_y y t_y \end{aligned} \quad [2.15a–c]$$

The amplitude of the echo reflects both the spin density and the phase dispersion. This is described by:

$$S(k_y) = \int \rho(y) \exp(-i 2\pi k_y y) dy \quad [2.16]$$

where:

$$k_y = \gamma G_y t_y / 2\pi \quad [2.17]$$

and k_y is a spatial frequency and has units of m^{-1}. For each value of the gradient, G_y, a single point in the two-dimensional array is essentially obtained. The full spatial frequency spectrum, $S(k_y)$, is obtained by changing the G_y gradient in small increments; if 2N+1 increments (commonly 128 or 256) are used, the signal becomes:

$$s\left(k_y\right) = \sum_{-N}^{N} \rho(y)\exp\left(-i2\pi k_{y1n}y\right) \qquad [2.18]$$

An inverse Fourier transform of $S(k_y)$ provides the spin density of $\rho(y)$.

Frequency Encoding

The influence of a linear gradient on the precession frequency is used to encode the spatial distribution of spin density. If a gradient is applied during a spin echo, the signal is written as:

$$S(k_x) = \int \rho(x)\exp(-i2\pi k_x x)dx \qquad [2.19]$$

where k_x is the spatial frequency in the direction of the frequency encode gradient (x-direction in this book). Note that the frequencies in frequency encoding are acquired all at once without repetition of the pulse sequence.

Combination of phase and frequency encoding results in a two-dimensional array of signal values with different k_y and k_x indices. A two-dimensional inverse Fourier transform yields the spin density as a function of x and y. When combined with a slice selection, all three coordinates are specified and a plane is imaged. A more detailed analysis of this experiment (Maneval, McCarthy & Whitaker 1990) shows that in reality the signal is modified by a relaxation time weighting:

$$S(k_x,k_y) = \int\int \rho(x,y)\exp[-TE/T_2]\exp[-i2\pi k_x/(\gamma G T_2)] \\ *\exp[-i2\pi(k_x x+k_y y)]dxdy \qquad [2.20]$$

Consequently, in order to obtain a true density image, the effects of relaxation times must be either removed or minimized to the point of insignificance. The signal can be corrected for relaxation time effects by acquiring a set of images with varying TE values to produce estimates of localized spin-spin relaxation times and local density values (Haacke, Liang & Tkach 1988; McCarthy 1990).

Fourier Imaging

The combination of slice selection, phase encoding, and frequency encoding in a basic spin echo pulse sequence is commonly referred to as Fourier imaging or spin-warp imaging. The basic pulse sequence detailing this combination is illustrated in Figure 1.4. The image information is reconstructed by using a two-dimensional Fourier transform of the data. Before Fourier transforming, the data set is usually corrected for any DC offsets by baseline correction and multiplied by a trapezoidal filter to minimize the effect of finite data set size.

Fourier imaging experiments are popular because the influence of spin-spin relaxation and spin-lattice relaxation is easily incorporated. Additionally, for spectrometers without shielded gradients, sufficient time can be designed into the experiment to allow the majority of eddy currents to decay prior to data acquisition.

Echo-Planar Imaging

Echo-planar imaging is a rapid method of Fourier imaging in which all of the information necessary for reconstruction of the image is acquired during one decay of the NMR signal. The spatial encoding is accomplished by using gradient recalled echoes and a weak constant field gradient. A gradient recalled echo is similar to a spin echo except that the refocusing is accomplished by reversing the direction of the magnetic field gradient. The advantage of echo-planar imaging is that a two-dimensional image can be acquired in less than 50 ms, allowing very rapid processes to be studied. Some of the disadvantages include a reduced signal-to-noise ratio and lower spatial resolution.

Projection Reconstruction

Lauterbur introduced this technique which was one of the first used to generate images (Lauterbur 1973). This method of image reconstruction is similar to that used in X-ray tomography. A series of one-dimensional projections, each acquired at a different angle of rotation about the sample, is used to reconstruct the image. There are a large number of algorithms for reconstruction of the image. The simplest is the back-projection method where the intensity of the profile is averaged back towards the direction of the original angle. This provides an image with artifacts from the projection procedure. By use of filters, artifacts are significantly reduced and the back-projection method can produce excellent representations of the original object.

Interpretation of Spin-Warp Imaging Signals

Information Content of NMR Image

The information in a given NMR signal can be influenced by experimental parameters, the design of the pulse sequence, and sample characteristics. As measured in an NMR experiment, the saturation of a component is actually nuclei density per a specific volume element. The volume element is defined by the pulse sequence applied and by the characteristics of the sample. If a static system is being imaged, the volume from which the signal is derived can be calculated by an analysis of the Bloch equation (Maneval, McCarthy & Whitaker 1990).

The nuclei density per unit volume is actually an integration over the sample. For instance, in a one-dimensional spatial image the signal is given by:

$$S(x) = \int_{x_1}^{x_2} \rho(x)dx \qquad [2.21]$$

For a two-dimensional spatial image, a double integration in space is performed. Thus, the information obtained has a characteristic length scale associated with the integration.

The length scale of the NMR measurement influences the information content of the NMR image. For example, in a flow imaging experiment where the spatial dimensions of each voxel are large compared to the extent of a no-slip region near a solid boundary, the no-slip region may not be apparent in the final data set. This occurs because the velocity is an average over all the velocities in the voxel and hence will give a non-zero value even for a voxel containing some fluid with a zero velocity.

Comparison of NMR Image Data to Theoretical Models

Basis of Theoretical Models

The calculation of the voxel dimensions for saturation measurements is critical when the results from the MRI experiment are to be compared with theoretical predictions. A theoretical analysis of transport processes in heterogeneous systems has two goals:

1. Define the form of the governing averaged equations for describing transport of energy, mass, and momentum.
2. Provide methods to predict the values of the effective transport coefficients in the governing equations.

Central to achieving both goals is the identification of the length and time scales important in both the averaged governing equations and the prediction of coefficients.

A dependent variable (concentration, temperature, velocity, or pressure) can be defined by using a volume averaging approach (Whitaker 1967):

$$\langle \Psi_\alpha \rangle(\mathbf{x}) = (1/V)\int \Psi_\alpha(\mathbf{y})dy \qquad [2.22]$$

where Ψ_α is the point value of the dependent variable, $\langle\Psi_\alpha\rangle(\mathbf{x})$ is the average of the point values of Ψ_α in the volume, V, centered at **x**. The new value, $\langle\Psi_\alpha\rangle(\mathbf{x})$, has a characteristic length scale of the averaging volume that is distinctly different from the length scale associated with the point value, Ψ_α. This process serves to give a smoothed value to the dependent variable.

A different mathematical description of the volume average of a dependent variable by use of a weight function (Marle 1982) is helpful for interpreting MRI measurements. In the weight function approach, the average point value is calculated by convolution of Ψ_α with a weight function, m(**y**). The value of the weight function is dependent only on the distance between the points **x** and **y**:

$$\langle\Psi_\alpha\rangle(\mathbf{x}) = \int \Psi_\alpha(\mathbf{y}) m(\mathbf{x}+\mathbf{y}) dy \qquad [2.23]$$

To make this approach useful, the characteristics of the weight function need to be defined. By this definition, the connection to the physical system is made. The next step is to relate experimental measurements to dependent variables.

Mathematical Basis for Comparison

The NMR spectrometer and sample used in an experiment produces a voltage that is proportional to some dependent variable, for example, nuclei density or velocity. For an NMR experiment, the weight function is given a physical meaning, for example, in terms of a spatial distribution of the signal recorded. In the specific case of using a spin-warp imaging pulse sequence for measuring moisture saturation, the weight function is:

$$m(\xi) = m_{sp}(\xi_1) m_{fe}(\xi_2) m_{pe}(\xi_3) \qquad [2.24]$$

where sp is selective pulse, fe is frequency encode, and pe is phase encode. The individual components of weight function are given in Table 2.1. Each weight function provides the length scale of the NMR measurement in a specific direction. Combined, they provide the information necessary for comparing the length scale of the measurement to the length scale of the theoretical model of the process (Maneval, McCarthy & Whitaker 1990).

Table 2.1. Spin-warp imaging weight functions.

slice selection	$m_{sp}(\xi_1)$	λ_{sp} = **slice thickness**
phase encode	$m_{fe}(\xi_2)$	$\lambda_{pe} = L/(N-1)$
frequence encode	$m_{pe}(\xi_3)$	$\lambda_{fe} = 1/\gamma G_{fe} T_2$

References

Belton, P. S., & Hills, B. P. 1987. The effects of diffusive exchange in heterogeneous systems on NMR line shapes and relaxation processes. *Molecular Physics* **61**: 999–1018.

Bloch, F. 1946. Nuclear induction. *Physical Review* **70**: 460–474.

Carr, H. Y., & Purcell, E. M. 1954. Effects of diffusion on free precession in nuclear magnetic resonance experiments. *Physical Review* **94**: 630–638.

Fukushima, E., & Roeder, S. B. W. 1981. *Experimental pulse NMR: A nuts and bolts approach*. New York: Addison-Wesley.

Haacke, E. M., Liang, Z.-P., & Tkach, J. A. 1988. T2-Deconvolution in MR imaging and spectroscopy. *J. of Magnetic Resonance* **76**: 440–457.

Hahn, E. L. 1950. Spin echoes. *Physical Review* **80**: 580–594.

Lauterbur, P. C. 1973. Image formation by induced local interactions: Examples employing nuclear magnetic resonance. *Nature* **242**: 190–191.

Maneval, J. E., McCarthy, M. J., & Whitaker, S. 1990. Use of nuclear magnetic resonance as an experimental probe in multiphase systems: Determination of the instrument weight function for measurements of liquid-phase volume fractions. *Water Resources Research* **26**: 2807–2816.

Marle, C. E. 1982. On macroscopic equations governing multiphase flow with diffusion and chemical reaction in porous media. *Int. J. Engng. Sci.* **20**: 643–662.

McCarthy, M. J. 1990. Interpretation of the magnetic resonance imaging signal from a foam. *AIChE J.* **36**: 287–290.

Morris, P. G. 1986. *Nuclear Magnetic Resonance Imaging in Medicine and Biology*. New York: Oxford University Press.

Whitaker, S. 1967. Diffusion and dispersion in porous media. *AIChE J.* **13**: 420–427.

3

Measurement of Food Structure and Component Functionality

Structure Measurement

Magnetic resonance imaging is capable of measuring structural features as well as the influence of processing, storage, and variations in formulation on the development of structural features. Strategies for measuring food structure using MRI and procedures for analyzing this information are presented here. MRI has the ability to measure certain structural features that cannot be measured by other experimental techniques, for example, the gas phase volume fraction as a function of position within a foam during formation of the foam (Philhofer 1992).

Experimental Setup

Design of an experiment to measure food structure needs to include considerations for the spectrometer (field shimming, RF pulse lengths) and the simulated process or storage container.

Probe

An NMR probe is most often considered to be only the electrical components and the materials necessary for physical support of the components and sample. However, for MRI of nonmedical samples, the electrical components often become a part of the simulated storage chamber or simulated process equipment. The advantages of combining the two are that the signal-to-noise ratio can be maximized and the probe configuration optimized for the particular process. For purposes of this discussion, the electrical components will be considered as separate from the sample chamber to the extent that the interaction between the two items is minimal with respect to the intended function of each item.

Common types of probe configurations for MRI include a surface coil, a birdcage coil, and a solenoid (single) coil. Simplified schematic diagrams of two of these configurations are shown in Figure 3.1; the single coil configuration is diagrammed in Figure 1.2.

The performance of the probe is influenced by several factors, for example, changes in temperature, sample changes, and nonlinear response. Both home-built and commercial probes generally operate well near room temperature. However, during food processing or storage studies, the temperature can vary dramatically over the course of an experiment. This can cause the characteristics of the electrical probe circuit to change and hence the tuning of the probe may vary during an experiment. If quantitative data is to be obtained, the probe electrical circuit needs to be maintained at a constant temperature or the NMR signal needs to be corrected for changes during the experiment. If the sample changes dramatically during an experiment even when the temperature remains constant, the resonant frequency and impedance matching of the probe can change. Appropriate safeguards to ensure accurate data are to measure the tuning of the probe before and after the experiment and, in extreme cases, to run the experiment and continuously monitor the probe resonant frequency and impedance.

Most NMR probes are assumed to have a uniform RF excitation field and a uniform RF response to the NMR signal. However, MRI probes frequently have a nonuniform response over the volume of interest. The method for correcting the signal is to measure the nonuniform response and to correct the final signal from an experiment using the measured nonuniform response. The nonlinear response of the probe is most easily measured by placing a homogeneous sample in the probe and recording the signal. Variations in the signal from the uniform sample then directly provide a map of the nonlinear response of the probe. This nonlinear response is analogous to the influence of a bad camera lens on a photograph, i.e., the image is distorted. In both cases, the correction procedure is the same: since the receiver coil response is convoluted with the MRI signal in the time domain, a simple division in the frequency domain corrects the signal intensity (McCarthy 1990; Turney 1990). However, this approach applies only to slight deviations; if the response of a coil varies by more than 10% across the sample, the probe should be modified.

Sample Container

Generally, sample containers can be of any construction as long as three constraints are met: (1) the container is not magnetic or paramagnetic, (2) metal is used sparingly and does not cover any portion of the sample being examined, and (3) the sample container fits inside the electronic probe. Plastics and ceramics are the best materials for the construction of sample containers. The construction material should be tested to determine if it has a detectable NMR signal.

The analysis of data from a particular experiment can often be greatly simplified by the design of the sample container. MRI data sets are typically large and require

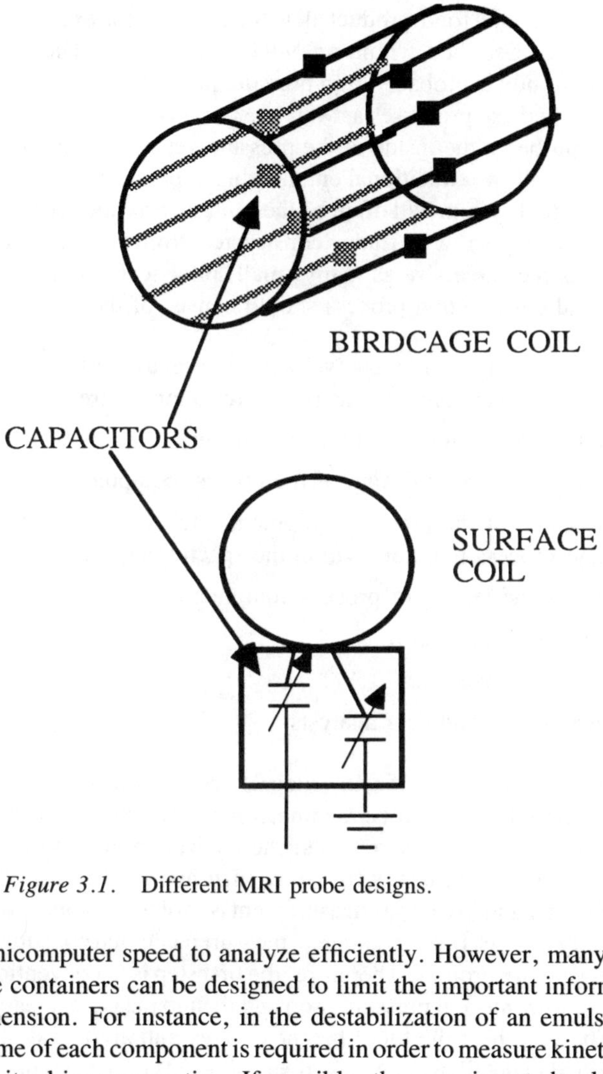

Figure 3.1. Different MRI probe designs.

at least minicomputer speed to analyze efficiently. However, many experiments and sample containers can be designed to limit the important information to one spatial dimension. For instance, in the destabilization of an emulsion, only the phase volume of each component is required in order to measure kinetic parameters of this gravity driven separation. If possible, the experiment should be set up to measure changes as a function of one spatial direction (height or width). This reduces the amount of data to be transferred, analyzed, and stored by two orders of magnitude. The disadvantage of one-dimensional data is that the images are not as visually striking as two-dimensional and three-dimensional images.

Process Equipment

The ability to use MRI to study the transport of heat, mass, and momentum within foods in simulated process equipment is perhaps the greatest new asset for food researchers and food product developers. Almost every food process can be simulated and studied within an MRI spectrometer. The most difficult type of process to study is probably high pressure processing. However, it should be possible to study these processes as well by specially constructing the gradient coils and NMR probe on the inside of the pressure vessel. Design of the process equipment should follow a traditional engineering approach for scaling down the process. The eventual system will often be the same size as pilot-scale equipment. For example, a single-screw extruder constructed from plastic with a 30 mm diameter barrel is the same size as many small, pilot-scale extruders.

The design and construction process should consist of the following steps:

1. Identification of the parameters (velocity, concentration) to be measured by MRI and conventional means (pressure, temperature)
2. Detailed simulation of data and data analysis
3. Preliminary engineering design of the process equipment
4. Detailed design of the process equipment, including layout to scale of motors and process monitors within the spectrometer room
5. Construction and testing of process equipment
6. Preliminary experimental runs
7. Modifications as necessary
8. Experimental runs and data analysis

The construction and utilization of a flow loop designed as a tube rheometer demonstrates some important steps. A tube rheometer measures volumetric flow rate and pressure drop. From these measurements, rheological properties of the fluid are determined, for example, viscosity for Newtonian fluids. The goal of the design of the tube rheometer and MRI flow measurement is to obtain comparisons between predicted velocity profiles from rheological measurements and constitutive models with measured velocity profiles. Therefore, the first step is to conventionally measure volumetric flow rate and pressure drop and then to measure a velocity profile using MRI. The design of the tube rheometer is essentially a scale-up problem which is described in detail by K. McCarthy et al. (1991). The essential feature of the rheometer is to ensure a fully developed flow between the pressure measuring devices. Fully developed flow is ensured by having a length-to-diameter ratio greater than 150 upstream of the first pressure measurement.

Detailed layout of the apparatus within the spectrometer room is needed in order to prevent interference between the equipment and the spectrometer. Interference can occur between equipment and fringe magnetic fields emanating from the magnet. For example, a wide-bore (45 cm), 2-tesla magnet may have a 5-gauss line of greater than 50 feet in diameter. Many measuring devices are susceptible to failure in low magnetic fields (5–10 gauss) and need to be kept a specific distance from the magnet. Motors must be kept out of the 50-gauss line or they may fail to operate. At this stage of the design process, the magnetic field plots listed in the magnet installation manual and vendor information on measuring devices must be consulted. When in doubt about the fabrication/operation of a measuring device, assume the worst case and maintain the item outside the 1-gauss line. The reason for this extreme caution is that it can be very costly and time-consuming to remove an item pulled into the magnet. More important, however, is the fact that an item pulled into a strong super-conducting magnet is accelerated to a high rate of speed as it approaches the magnet. Anyone between the magnet and the moving object can be seriously hurt.

Another consideration at this stage is the setup of the simulation before operation. Normally, the simulated process must be like a large tinker toy, i.e., easy to break down into smaller, easily moved pieces. This facilitates transfer of the equipment into and out of the spectrometer room. The setup, however, must be done in such a way that normal tools (such as iron wrenches, screwdrivers, etc.) are not used because of the close proximity to the magnetic field. If necessary, special nonmagnetic wrenches can be purchased or fabricated for the setup and breakdown phases. Usually the system can be designed with plastic fittings that can be hand-tightened or tightened with a wrench outside the 5-gauss field line and then installed.

At this point, the construction and testing of the process equipment should be straightforward and is essentially a job for a mechanical shop. The electrical probe should also be built at this time or tested to ensure that it will function with the device. This is trivial for a tube rheometer; however, for other process simulation situations, it may be quite difficult. For example, the initial designs of a single-screw extruder had to be modified in order to compensate for the electrical components of the probe. Testing of the equipment is similar to that for any type of research or pilot-scale system. In one particular instance when a tube rheometer was used, homogeneous pure fluids were characterized on laboratory rheometers and the measurements compared to those obtained from the newly-constructed system. Very good agreement between the rheological parameters was obtained. Preliminary experimental results were also very good. However, a 60 Hz artifact was seen in every image. This was probably due to the discrete nature of the flow from the gear pump or else by the vibration in the tubing induced by the pump. A flexible connection was installed and the artifact was significantly reduced.

Spectrometer Setup

All precautions/setups for standard NMR spectrometers should be followed. However, two items—the homogeneity of the field and the setting of the initial 90° pulse strength—have deviations from standard spectroscopy. The field homogeneity for imaging (with the exception of chemical shift imaging) does not need to be as good as for high-resolution spectroscopy. This is because a gradient is used to degrade the uniformity of the field in order to encode spatial information. Thus, the amount of time spent shimming the field can usually be significantly reduced. For instance, shimming on a pure water sample until the line is on the order of several Hz will not alter the image quality if the original line width was on the order of 20–30 Hz. With semisolid materials, the best approach to shimming is often to just turn off the room temperature shim set. The second aspect that is different from standard spectroscopy is setting the pulse power of a selective 90° pulse. Care should be taken to maximize the signal after this pulse since the magnitude of the free induction decay (which is a maximum for a 90° rotation) is being observed. This is often not clearly stated in manuals and it is often overlooked in initial studies by individuals learning MRI techniques.

Shielded Gradients

The rapid switching of linear magnetic field gradients during an MRI experiment can result in distortion of the signal from the sample. This distortion arises from additional fluctuating magnetic fields in the conducting structures within the bore of the magnet. The fluctuating magnetic fields are generated from eddy currents within the conducting structures and oppose the fields generated during gradient switching. These fluctuating magnetic fields within the metal structures induce an alternating current in the inductor of the NMR probe and are recorded during data acquisition along with the NMR signal.

Shielded gradients were developed in order to reduce the magnitude and duration of eddy currents and to thereby minimize experimental artifacts. Eddy currents are reduced by designing the gradient coil to generate magnetic fields only inside the bore of the superconducting magnet. This is accomplished by using an additional set of gradient coils. These coils are specifically designed to cancel the magnetic field of the inner coils that is directed toward the cryostat, and to not influence the magnetic fields across the sample. The overall advantages of this type of system are faster rise times, good linearity in the applied field, and rapid decay of residual gradient fields. Almost all imaging experiments will have improved performance if shielded gradients are used instead of conventional unshielded gradients. However, in many cases the improvement is difficult to quantify since it is almost unmeasurable. The author recommends purchasing a system with shielded gradients or upgrading to shielded gradients whenever possible.

If shielded gradients are not available, there are many ways to work around or to minimize the influence of eddy currents. The first is to determine if the pre-emphasis of the gradient waveforms is operating properly and if the gradient amplifiers are operating properly. This includes reviewing electrical connections between the gradient amplifiers and the gradient coils. Frequently, gradient performance can be improved by shortening the length of the connecting cables. After reviewing the hardware, pulse sequences can be used to allow data acquisition long after gradient pulses. One way is to use a stimulated echo experiment to measure diffusion as opposed to using a spin-echo experiment; another way is to alter the shape of the gradient in order to minimize eddy currents (Majors et al. 1990). The author has worked exclusively on MRI spectrometers without shielded gradients. The only experiments that have proven unacceptable have been echo planar imaging, some gradient recalled imaging, and a few spin-echo-based diffusion measurements. However, many hours have been spent working to minimize the effects of eddy currents.

Analysis of NMR Signal

MRI can provide temporal and spatial information at previously unavailable spatial and temporal densities. However, converting this information into a useful form can be a difficult task because the experimenter must remember that all NMR properties can depend upon spatial position and time.

Phase Volume Measurements/Concentrations

The NMR signal is essentially a measure of nuclei density per volume. This nuclei density is usually calibrated by comparison to a standard reference. For example, a standard reference for hydrogen could be a vial of water of known volume. The signal from an unknown would then be compared to the reference standard and the ratio would provide an accurate value of the proton density in the unknown.

This comparison and measuring of a quantity using standard high-resolution or low-resolution techniques is straightforward. However, attempting to measure changes in concentration using spatially resolved measurement is more difficult. Several factors need to be considered:

1. Spatial alignment of the sample and gradients
2. Influence of variations in NMR parameters and sample heterogeneity
3. Length scale of the NMR measurement

In discussing the influence of these factors, we assume that the effective spin-spin relaxation time does not control spatial resolution in the frequency encode direction, and that the selective pulse excites a well-defined plane. Additionally, the factors are discussed for spatial encoding in only one direction (the frequency encode direction). The extension of the discussion to two and three dimensions is straightforward (with the additional complexities of geometry).

Ensuring that the sample and gradients are aligned is important for quantitative studies. Errors can occur in calculation of concentration gradients if the sample and gradients are not aligned. Consider a rectangular container aligned parallel to the direction of gravity. If the linear gradient in the direction of gravity (say X-gradient) is rotated 5° clockwise compared to the gravity vector, a one-dimensional projection results that is different than expected. This can easily occur if the spectrometer is not set up correctly or if the sample is not correctly aligned.

The next factor of importance is a change in one of the material properties, either NMR relaxation times or material heterogeneity. NMR relaxation times can depend on phase concentrations. For unknown samples, the variation of relaxation time with position and phase volume should be measured to determine if this is important. Procedures for correcting the signal intensity for variations in relaxation times will be presented later in this chapter. If relaxation times do not vary significantly over wide changes in concentration, one still must be concerned with changes in solids content per unit volume.

Most food materials shrink during drying and this results in an increase of the solids concentration at the drying surface. The change in the NMR signal reflects only a decrease in mobile nuclei per unit volume and, in general, provides no information on changes in solids concentration. Unless the rate and the spatial dependence of shrinkage is known, errors will occur in converting nuclei per unit volume into phase amount per amount of dry solids. Procedures for correcting the signal intensity in such cases are outlined in Chapter 5.

Dynamics

When the dynamics of a process or change is to be measured, the time for acquiring an image must be less than the time over which a measurable change occurs. A standard spin-echo image can be acquired in approximately 5–10 minutes. This time scale is adequate to quantify dynamic changes for many systems. In the case of drying of agricultural materials, the process occurs over several hours to several days and hence an image every 5 minutes is adequate to describe changes. However, 5 minutes is inadequate to quantify rapid changes such as the collapse of foam on an American beer. Two approaches exist to quantify this type of dynamic behavior. The first is to reduce the process to a 1-D process in which the information can be acquired in 1 second or less. The other is to use a rapid imaging technique such as echo planar imaging.

Flow Measurements

MRI is becoming one of the premier methods for flow visualization and measurement. The two basic types of MRI flow measurement techniques are time-of-flight methods and phase encoding methods.

Time-of-flight methods are based on exciting the spins in one position and recording their position at a later time. This is demonstrated for the case of plug flow in Figure 3.2. Variations on this basic flow measurement include offsetting the plane of tagging for flow parallel to the direction of tagging or incrementing a delay time for flow perpendicular to the slice selection gradient.

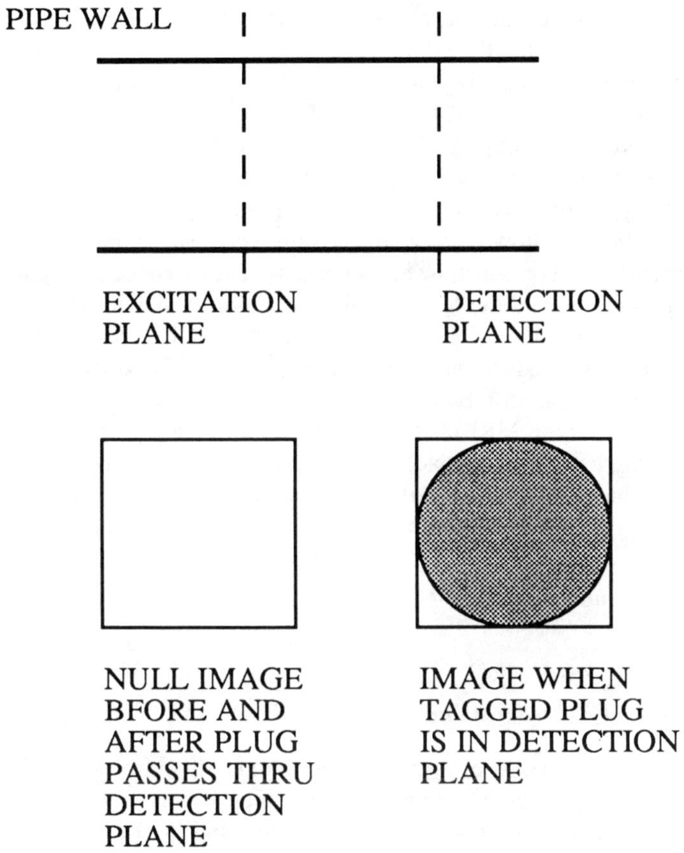

Figure 3.2. Time-of-flight detection for plug flow.

Phase encoding is based on measuring a small displacement parallel to a linear field gradient by the influence of the displacement on the phase of the NMR signal. For coherent (bulk) motion of a spin, the displacement, $\mathbf{r}$(t), is given by:

$$\mathbf{r}(t) = \mathbf{r}_0 + \mathbf{v}t \quad [3.1]$$

where $\mathbf{r}_0$ is the initial position of the spin at time zero and $\mathbf{v}$ is the velocity of the spin. If the spin moves at a constant velocity, v_z, in the direction of a field gradient, it will acquire a phase angle in proportion to its motion. To see this, the Bloch equations along with the above equation are used to give:

$$\phi = \gamma \int \mathrm{G}\cdot\mathbf{r}\, dt \quad [3.2]$$

$$\phi = \gamma(r_0 m_0 + \nu\, m_1) \quad [3.3]$$

where ϕ is the phase, and m_0 and m_1 are the zeroth and first moments of the gradient waveform in the time domain. If the gradient is designed in such a way that $m_0 = 0$ but $m_1 \neq 0$, this phase angle will be proportional to the velocity of the spin. Just as the phase of the magnetization was used to measure the spin density distribution, a properly designed gradient allows the phase to be used to measure the distribution of velocities in a sample.

For both types of flow measurements, it is important to remember that the signal proportional to flow is an average within each voxel. The averaging process is different for both types of flow measurement. The extent of averaging depends on the type of flow and the length scales of the measurement and the process. For example, in the flow of paper pulp suspensions it is expected that a 3% by weight mixture will exhibit plug flow. This plug flow of paper pulp also has a very thin layer of almost pure water at the surface of the pipe, the no-slip boundary layer. When MRI phase encoded velocity measurements are taken in which the length scale of a voxel is much greater than the thickness of the no-slip region, the no-slip region will not be detected, as is shown in Figure 3.3. Analysis of MRI velocity encoding is an active area of research.

Examples of Food Structure Measurement

Foams

Experimental Procedures and Data Analysis

A foam is a dispersion of a gas in a continuous liquid or solid phase. Only the analysis of liquid/gas foams will be presented in this section. Typical food foams are whipped egg whites, whipped cream, and the head on beer. Liquid foams are thermodynamically unstable systems and tend toward collapse. The mechanism for collapse is the loss of liquid between bubbles. This results from liquid drainage caused by gravity and by stress induced by gas diffusion between bubbles. Evaporation can also play an important role in reducing liquid between the gas phase bubbles. Methods to stabilize foams center on increasing the viscosity in order to slow liquid drainage and increasing the stability of the gas-liquid interface in order to delay breakage.

The complex nature of foams results in systems that are difficult to characterize. For instance, how can the bubbles in foam be measured without altering the bubbles? MRI techniques can assist in acquiring such new information about foams as phase volumes as a function of position, liquid drainage rates derived from phase volume data, rate of foam collapse, and cling.

Phase Volume

The constituents of a foam fall into three categories: the gas phase, solvent (typically water), and macromolecules (proteins, lipids, etc.). During MRI, sig-

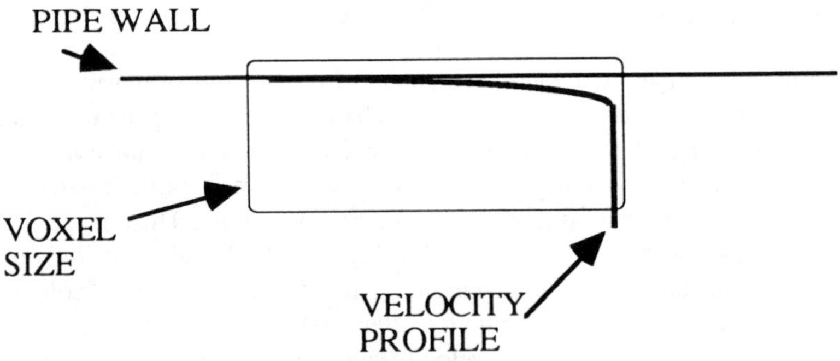

Figure 3.3. Example of where the voxel is large in one spatial dimension as compared to the high shear region of flow.

nals from macromolecules contribute either slightly or not at all to the signal and therefore they will not be considered in the following analysis. The goal of phase volume measurements is to quantify as a function of time the amount of liquid and gas at each position in the foam. A standard spin-echo-based Fourier imaging sequence with the phase encode gradient turned off will yield a signal of the following form:

$$S(x) = k\rho(x)(1-\exp(-TR/T_1(x))\exp(-TE/T_2(x)) \qquad [3.4]$$

If TR>>T_1, then the equation simply reduces to a T_2 weighting. The procedure for relating S(x) to a liquid density value includes the following steps:

1. Measure the signal intensity as a function of height for the completely filled container.
2. Vary the TE value for data acquisition or acquire multiple echoes for calculating T_2 values.

The first procedure is important in order to correct for variations in the response of the NMR probe. This essentially allows mapping of the constant of proportionality, k, as a function of height in the foam (in this case, X direction). After the data sets are corrected for nonlinear probe response, the intensity can be corrected for T_2 relaxation effects.

The procedure for correcting for the influence of variations in T_2 can be difficult to implement with a high degree of accuracy. This is because of two factors: First, many foams collapse fairly rapidly and can change over the time frame of a typical T_2 measurement; second, as the system drains, the signal-to-noise ratio decreases in the foam and therefore the accuracy of T_2 estimates decreases. For rapidly destabilizing foams, it is best to use a simple 90° pulse under the influence of a gradient in order to obtain the density profile; however, this can be a difficult experiment to implement with unshielded gradients.

Liquid Drainage

The liquid drainage rate can be calculated from a series of density profiles at different times. The drainage rate is the change in density per unit time. The time rate of change in the gas phase volume is related to the change in the liquid phase density. In most foams, some regions will have a constant density. This occurs because the liquid inflow equals the liquid outflow. The change in liquid density of egg white foam is illustrated in Figure 3.4. Signal intensity is proportional to liquid density. Overall height of the foam was 4 cm. Profiles were acquired at 1, 5, 7, 9, and 11 minutes after whipping.

Actual measurements of fluid velocity and fluid velocity profiles in a foam would be extremely difficult. The best approach may be to treat the system as a process of perfusion. The difficulty with perfusion imaging is that the results are hard to validate and are probably not specific for a particular model of flow.

Collapse

Collapse of a foam results from bubble wall rupture. This causes an overall decrease in the height of the foam column which is apparent in a decrease in the extent of spatial distribution in the MRI signal. As in the case of liquid drainage, a rate can be calculated from a series of MRI data sets. Collapse and drainage of a beer foam is shown in Figure 3.5.

Relaxation Effects

In a multiphase system such as foam, relaxation times will generally vary as the phase density varies (McCarthy 1990). However, this is not always the case (Assink et al. 1989); it is necessary to check to determine if variations in relaxation times exist. For foams, there are usually several effects in a spin echo-based sequence that influence the apparent T_2 value. Most prominent are the actual spin-spin relaxation times, the influence of magnetic susceptibility variations (13 ppm for an air-water interface), diffusion, and exchange. In a stable foam, it is usually possible to quantify the contributions from each of the phenomena influencing the decay of the spin echo signal. Thus, one possible method of estimating average bubble size is through analysis of susceptibility variations and the state of macromolecules at the air-solution interface.

Additional Applications

Solid foams such as cakes, cookies, and biscuits can also be studied using MRI. Both the mass transfer and the void distribution that occurs during the baking of a biscuit have been studied (Heil, Özilgen & McCarthy 1992). A difficulty with solid foams (Fig. 3.6) is that quantifying the density of a component is more difficult than it is with liquid foams. The solid (macromolecules) becomes a significant fraction of the system, and the moisture per unit of dry solids is

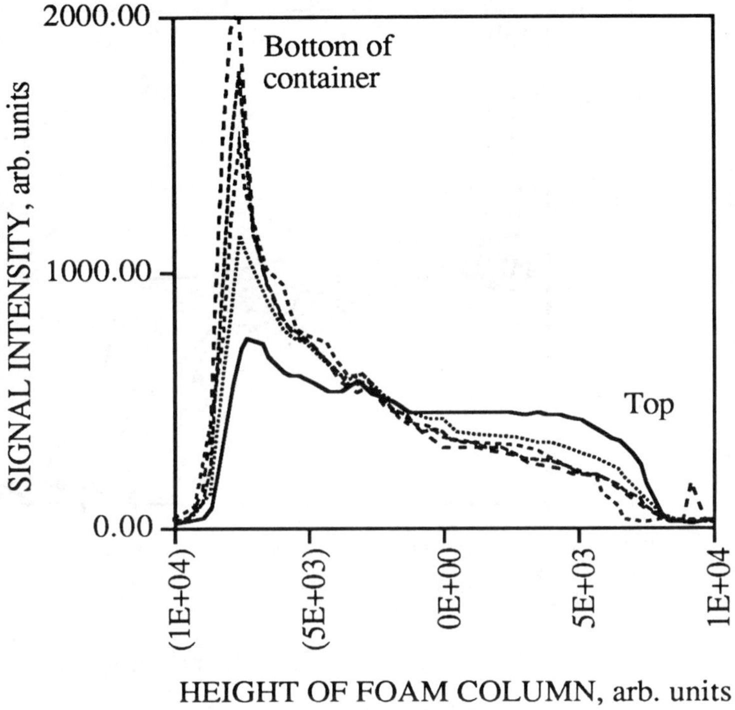

Figure 3.4. Liquid drainage in an egg white foam.

the quantity that is most useful for food scientists. However, standard MRI techniques provide information only on nuclei density per unit volume. The author knows of no precise method of conversion between the two values unless assumptions are made or an empirical relationship is developed. Frequently, only semiquantitative data is needed and/or if the biscuit structure is essentially uniform, a conversion to grams of moisture per gram of dry solids is possible (with an error as large as 10–15%).

More complex systems such as foamed emulsions (ice cream, for example) are more difficult to study. Using chemical shift imaging, the lipid, water, and air distributions can be determined. The disadvantage of chemical shift imaging is that additional time is required for the procedure and consequently only the more stable systems can be studied.

Emulsions

Experimental Procedures and Data Analysis

Phase Volume

The two approaches to measure phase volume as a function of position within an emulsion are direct and indirect. The direct approach is to use chemical shift imaging and integrate the areas in the spectra to provide a measurement of the

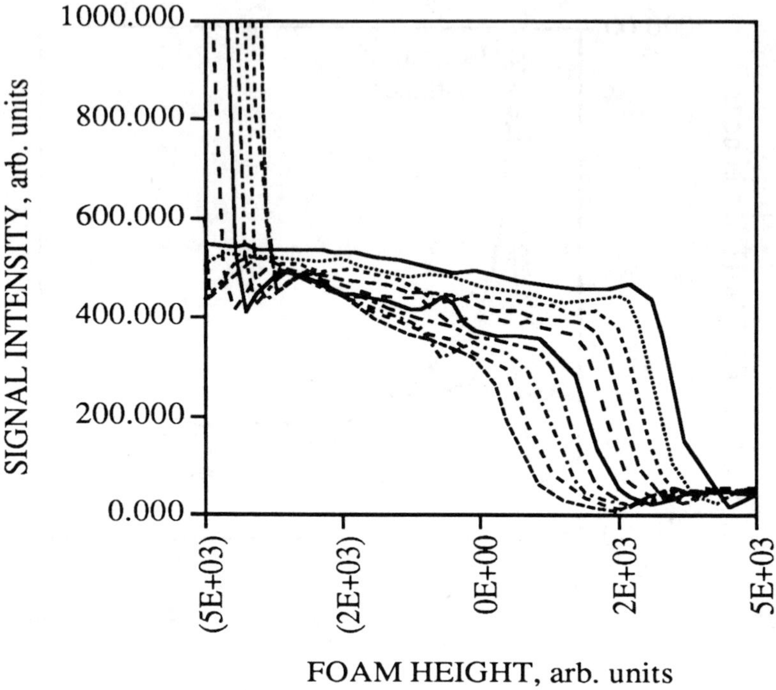

Figure 3.5. The collapse and drainage of a beer foam.

quantity of each phase. The indirect approach is to use the variation in an NMR parameter with concentration to make an indirect measurement. Examples of NMR parameters that are used include spin-lattice relaxation time and diffusivity.

Quantification of phase volumes using chemical shift imaging initially appears attractive because it is a direct measurement. However, there are several complications: Quantification is not easy, chemical shift imaging is time consuming, and the volume of data can be large. Quantification of phases in an emulsion requires a procedure similar to that used to measure foam drainage. First, a standard is characterized to determine if a nonuniform response exists. Care needs to be taken to correct for T_1 or T_2 relaxation time variations with concentration and species. A single point in a foam drainage study becomes a spectrum in an emulsion study. Therefore, the same difficulties of quantification for species in high-resolution NMR studies apply to the spectra in chemical shift imaging. In a chemical shift image, the spectral lines are frequently broader and overlap more than in a high-resolution spectra; this complicates the integration of areas. However, chemical shift imaging is the preferred method to measure phase volumes as a function of position. (Remember, of course, that since oil and water have slightly different resonant frequencies, a spatial misregistration between the two phases exists in MRI procedures.)

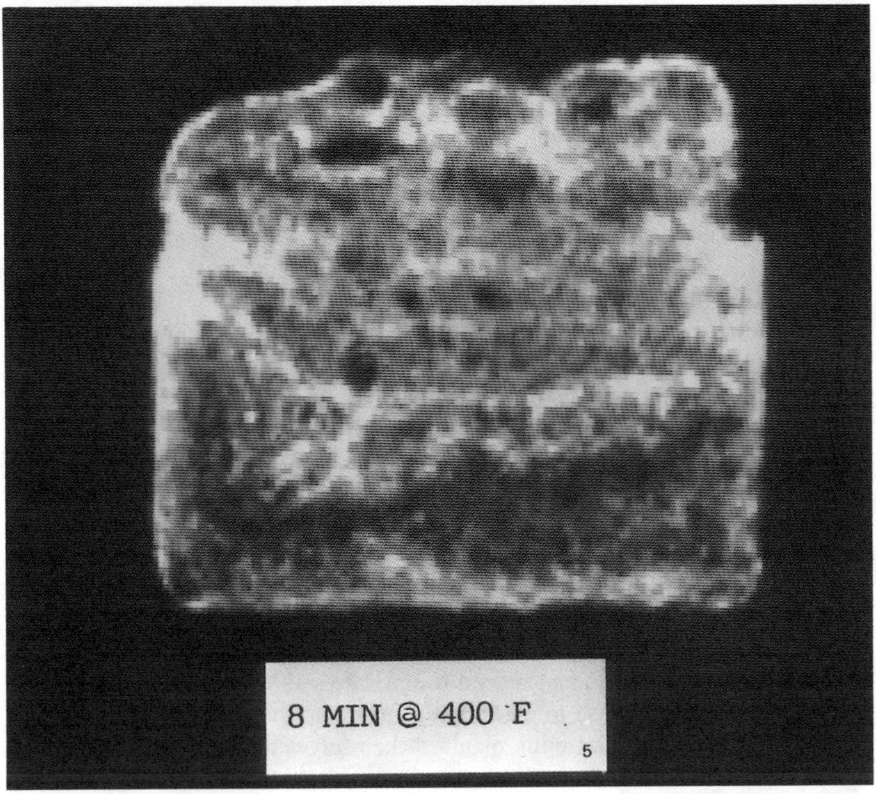

Figure 3.6. Proton density image of an American-style biscuit.

It is sometimes advantageous to use indirect methods to study destabilization in emulsions because the destabilization can be rapid, there may be significantly reduced amounts of data, and there is reduced complexity in data analysis compared to chemical shift imaging. One method of indirectly measuring phase volumes is using a two-point T_1 estimate (Kauten, Maneval & McCarthy 1991). In many emulsion systems, the T_1 of each phase is significantly different. Thus if a two-point T_1 estimate is made on the emulsion, an averaged value of T_1 for both phases is obtained. A ratio of the acquired signal intensities provides a T_1 estimate:

$$T_1 = \frac{-\tau}{\ln(1 - S_1/S_2)} \qquad [3.5]$$

The T_1 volume fraction relationship has been found (Kauten, Maneval & McCarthy 1991) to obey the simple equation:

$$\frac{1}{T_{1(obs)}} = \frac{\phi_{(1)}}{T_{1(1)}} + \frac{\phi_{(2)}}{T_{1(2)}} \qquad [3.6]$$

where ϕ is the phase fraction of component 1 or 2 and $T_{1(obs)}$ stands for observed T_1 value, $T_{1(1)}$ and $T_{1(2)}$ are the pure phase relaxation times. This relationship may not apply to all systems, particularly if the T_1s of each phase are not significantly different; if the phase volume of one phase is very small, slight errors in measurements will probably render the procedure useless.

Droplet Size Distribution

In addition to the concentration profile, the droplet size distribution is important to the functionality, texture, and stability of an emulsion product. Typical methods of measuring particle size distributions include light scattering, ultrasound, and pulsed field gradient NMR studies. The pulsed field gradient NMR techniques are based on the measurement of the effect of barriers on the diffusion coefficient measurement.

Beginning with the spin-echo studies of Hahn (1950), measurement and analysis of diffusion effects have had a long history in the NMR literature. More recent efforts have focused on the use of the pulsed field gradient (PFG) techniques (Callaghan 1984; Stilbs 1987) which were first introduced by Stejskal and Tanner (1965). The basic PFG sequence is similar in some respects to the sequences used to measure velocities and indeed it may be used as such. The focus here, however, will be on its use to measure diffusive motion.

The effects of coherent motion manifest themselves in the phase of the NMR signal. In contrast, the effects of incoherent motion manifest themselves in an irreversible attenuation of the signal amplitude. If a spin does not move during the pulse sequence, there is no net effect on the gradient pulses in the PFG sequence and the phase of the spin remains unchanged at the echo time. However, if the spin makes a random jump to a new position during the pulse sequence, the dephasing effect of the first gradient pulse is imperfectly compensated by the second pulse and there is a net phase angle for the spin at the echo time. By considering an ensemble of spins moving via a random process (e.g., Brownian motion), it is clear that diffusive motion will result in a distribution of phase angles at the echo time. Since the motion is irreversible, diffusive motion manifests itself as an irreversible attenuation of the echo, much the same as intrinsic T_2 relaxation would.

More rigorous analyses of the effects of diffusion on NMR echo heights are available (Carr & Purcell 1954; Stilbs 1987). Only the results are considered here. The extra attenuation brought about by diffusion in the PFG sequence is quantified by ratioing the echo height measured when $g \neq 0$ to that measured when $g = 0$. For liquids, this ratio is related to the parameters of the pulse sequence as:

$$R = \exp[-\gamma^2(\delta g)^2 D(\Delta - \delta/3)] \qquad [3.7]$$

where g is the magnitude of the applied gradient, δ is its duration, and Δ is the separation between the two gradient pulses. Measurement of R for several different gradient strengths or separations will give the diffusion coefficient from measurements of the slope of a semilogarithmic plot of R vs. Δ or g^2. A typical plot for water is shown in Figure 3.7.

If a sample has internal structure that can lead to spatial variations in the local diffusion coefficient in a sample, NMR imaging methods may be used to localize PFG measurements and thereby map out the diffusivities in a sample. The approach essentially grafts the PFG sequence onto the spin-warp imaging sequence to provide signals whose intensities are representative of local diffusive motion rather than local spin concentrations (Klammler & Kimmich 1990; Taylor & Bushell, 1985). Examples include measurement of diffusion coefficients in various portions of intact chicken eggs (Klammler & Kimmich 1990; Taylor & Bushell 1985) and the study of non-Newtonian flow in micro-capillaries (Xia & Callaghan 1990).

The measurements of observation time dependent diffusivities in materials has been used as a means of nondestructive estimation of sample structural characteristics. These so-called restricted-diffusion measurements were presented with the introduction of the PFG methods (Stejskal 1965; Tanner & Stejskal 1968) and many of their applications and techniques have been reviewed recently (Callaghan 1984; Kärger, Pfeifer & Heink 1988). For example, Packer and Rees (1972) and Callaghan, Jolley, and Humphrey (1983) used restricted-diffusion methods to estimate droplet size distributions in emulsions. Comparison with optical and photographic methods showed that NMR produced good results.

More recent applications of the restricted-diffusion measurements include pore-space connectivity estimation (so-called *q*-space imaging)(Callaghan et al. 1990; Packer & Zelaya, 1989); cell-size and compartmentation estimation (Cory & Garroway 1990); and catalyst characterization (Cheng, Luthra & Pereira 1990). By use of the diffusion coefficient, the restricted-diffusion methods hold the possibility of making less-than-image-resolution measurements on multiphase systems.

Additional Applications

Using a combination of phase volume measurement and droplet size distribution measurements would provide information on the mechanisms of emulsion destabilization. It should be possible to qualitatively separate the influence of flocculation and coalescence. If NMR procedures are combined with ultrasound, then flocculation and coalescence could be separately quantified.

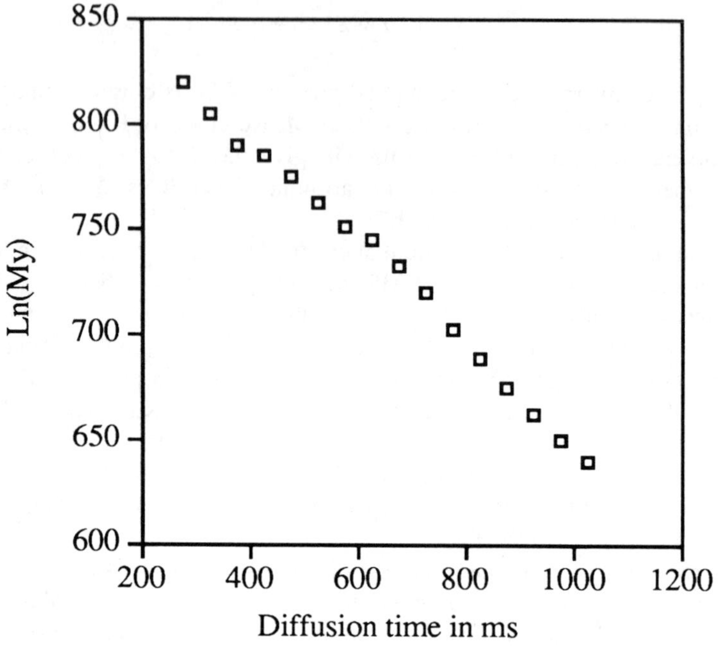

Figure 3.7. Echo attenuation as a function of diffusion time.

Suspensions

Improved characterization of the flow behavior and rheology of food suspensions should increase the efficiency of processing, improve product quality, and enhance the safety of fluid food products. Typical food suspensions are tomato juice, salad dressings, fruit juices, stews, and vegetable soups. At the present time, the rheology and fluid dynamics of these systems are generally not completely and accurately characterized. Additionally, those rheological characterizations that do exist are based on the assumption that the suspension has a well-defined flow field. However, this is not the case for many suspensions.

Experimental Procedures and Data Analysis

Velocity Measurements

The two basic methods to measure flow of materials using magnetic resonance are time-of-flight and phase encoding. Time-of-flight techniques rely on exciting the material at one location and, after a given time interval, detecting the excited spins at a different location. The velocity is then calculated from the change in position during the time interval. The excitation and detection for a typical time-of-flight technique is shown in Figure 3.8.

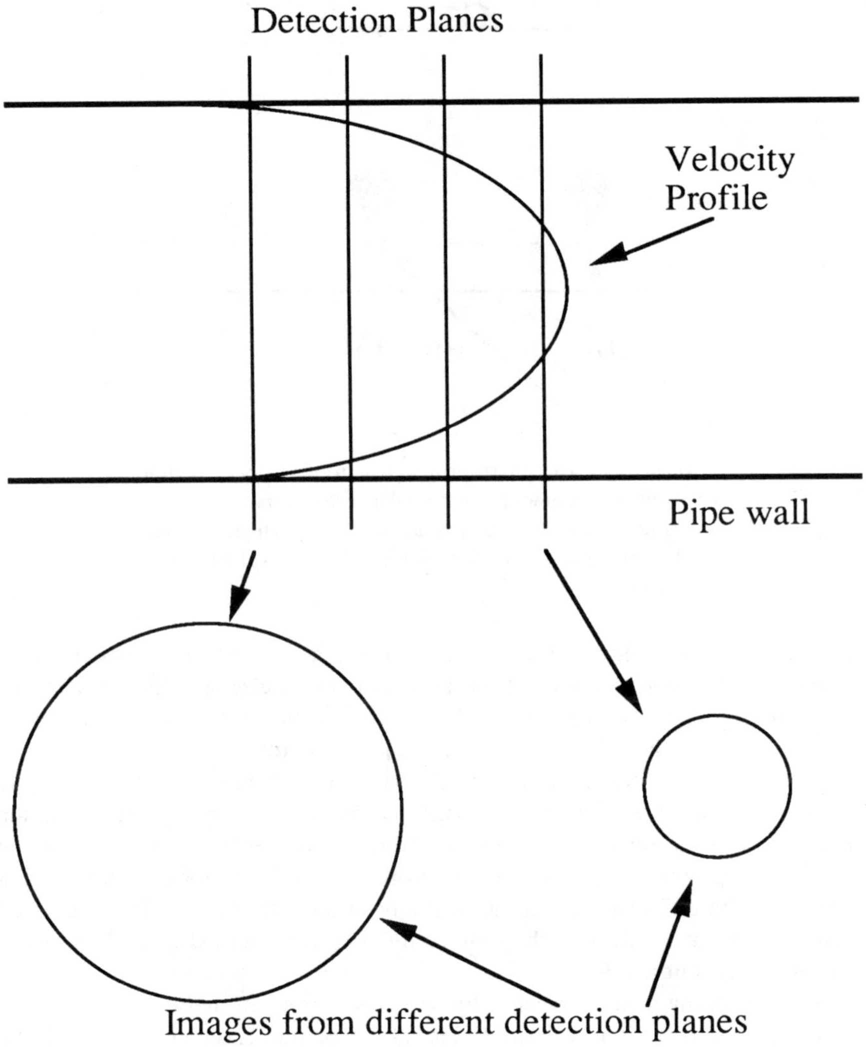

Figure 3.8. Time-of-flight flow measurements for laminar flow of a Newtonian fluid in a tube.

The second technique is termed *phase encoding* because the phase of the spins are made proportional to the velocity. This is accomplished by applying a linear field gradient in the direction of the velocity component of interest (detailed in Figure 3.9).

Time-of-flight (TOF) techniques are well suited for measuring flows in simple geometries of both complex and simple fluids and for measuring the flow of simple fluids in complex flow fields. TOF is not well suited for high velocity flows

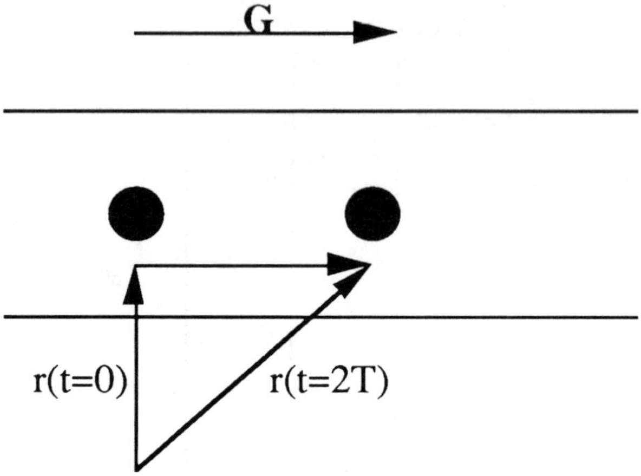

Figure 3.9. The phase of a signal from a packet of fluid (dark circle) becomes proportional to distance traveled during the time of the encoding gradient. Using an appropriate model, this distance is then converted into a velocity measurement.

or for nonrectilinear flows. A useful variation on the standard TOF experiment is to apply a 180° selective pulse prior to a spin-warp pulse sequence that results in the nulling of the signal from a plane. The displacement of the nulled plane directly maps out the velocity field in the object and provides an easy comparison with point velocity predictions from theory. The comparison should be made between the interface of the nulled plane and the plane of strong signal with the predictions of the mathematical model. Care should be taken in the design of the pulse sequence to eliminate any undesired flow effects, for example, during slice selection and phase encoding of the position. This type of TOF has been applied very successfully to the flow of fluids in a model extruder (McCarthy, Kauten & Agemura 1992).

Phase encoding is accomplished by applying a gradient in the direction along which flow information is desired. The effect of this gradient is to make the phase of the spins proportional to the velocity. The relationship is given by Equation 3.2. The form of the equation for the phase depends on the model used to describe the displacement of the spin. Higher order terms can be used to measure acceleration or jerk. The gradient waveforms are usually designed to encode the phase with only velocity information. This is performed by making the zeroth moment of the gradient waveform zero. Therefore, the only remaining term in Equation 3.3 is the term proportional to velocity. The pulse sequence is repeated for many different values of the gradient strength. This repetition process "sweeps out" the reciprocal domain for velocity. A Fourier transform of the data set will yield the velocity spectrum which is a histogram of the velocities in the sample. By application of a frequency encoding gradient during data acquisition, the velocity profile can be obtained directly. Figure 3.10 shows the application of this method to measure the velocity profile of a particulate suspension.

Analysis of MRI flow measurements becomes more complex in the flow of suspensions or flow in porous media. Procedures for analyzing the length scale of the measurement are well developed for static MRI imaging (Maneval, McCarthy & Whitaker 1990) and are under development for flow systems (McCarthy, Maneval & Powell 1992).

Rheological Information

Utilizing MRI velocity measurements to obtain information on the rheology of fluids is just beginning (Abbott et al. 1991; Sinton & Chow 1991; McCarthy, Maneval & Powell 1992). The author and co-workers have demonstrated that rheological parameters for simple fluids can be estimated with accuracy equivalent to standard rheometers. In addition to the rheological parameters, information on deviation from simple rheological model descriptions can be quantified.

Quantification of rheological parameters is outlined in the article by McCarthy,

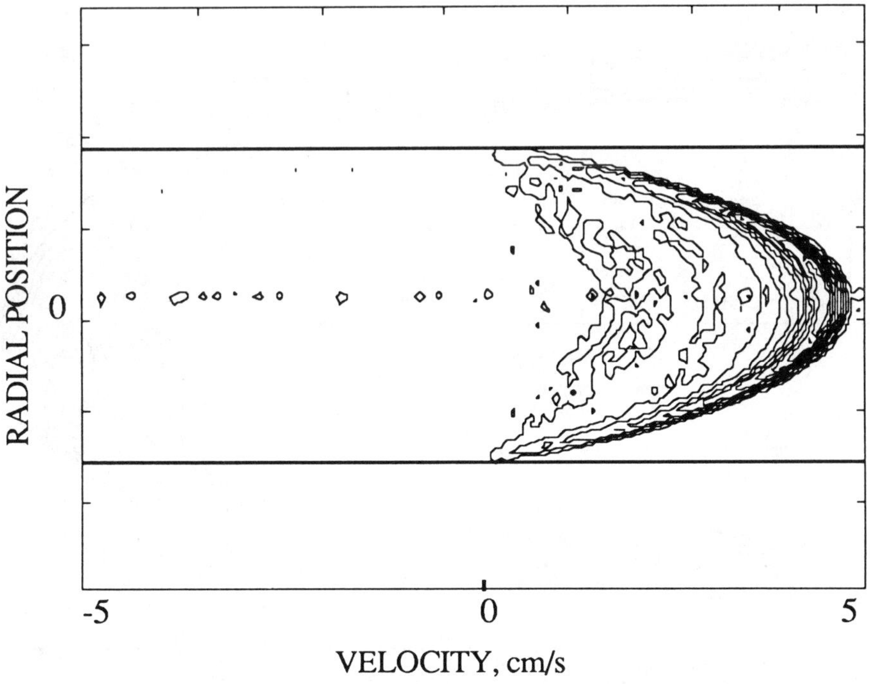

Figure 3.10. Joint spatial-velocity density distribution for particulate suspension (average velocity 0.0231 m/s, particle phase volume 36.2%, average radius 215μm).

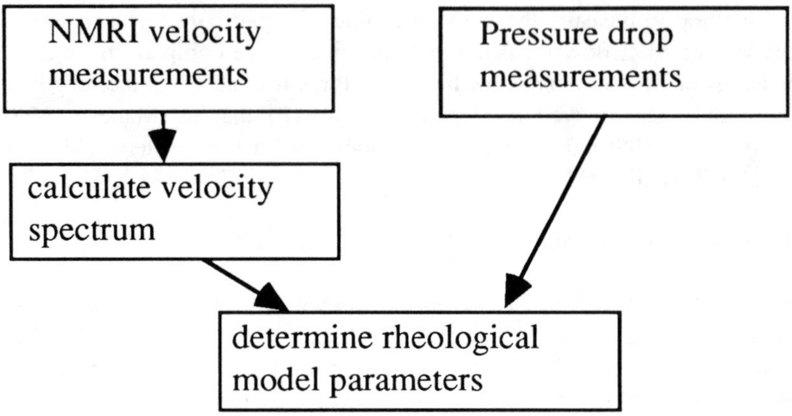

Figure 3.11. Steps in determining rheological properties using a measurement of the velocity spectrum.

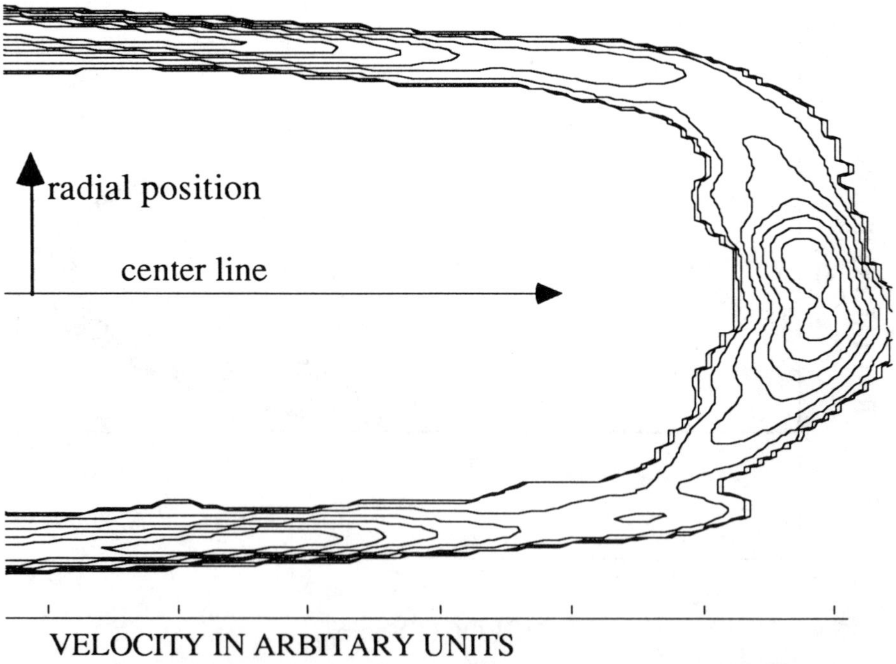

Figure 3.12. Contour plot of joint spatial-velocity density distribution function for water in tube flow (Reynolds number 4000, tube diameter 0.026 m).

Maneval and Powell (1992). The basic steps are to phase encode the flow, calculate the velocity spectrum (Fig. 3.11), and then convert this information into estimates of rheological parameters. For example, the value of n for a power-law fluid in laminar flow can be estimated from the value of the velocity spectrum at v = 0.

It is important to understand that the velocity spectrum has a unique relationship to the velocity profile for only simple flow fields such as laminar flow of a Newtonian liquid in a tube of circular cross-section. In more complex flow fields or geometries, there are many velocity profiles which could generate the same velocity spectrum (McCarthy, Maneval & Powell 1992).

Developments in applying flow imaging techniques to obtain rheological information are rapid. The reader should consult the recent literature for the most appropriate and efficient techniques.

Additional Applications

MRI flow measurements are providing significant new information on the rheology and fluid dynamics of opaque fluids and suspensions. Mixing, secondary flows, and turbulence (Fig. 3.12) can be studied in pure fluids and suspensions, particularly with the development of echo-planar flow imaging pulse sequences (Kose 1990). The potential also exists to study deformations in solid materials and MRI techniques may yield new information in the field of solid rheology.

References

Abbott, J. R., Tetlow, N., Graham, A. L., Altobelli, S. A., & Fukushima, E. 1991. Experimental observation of particle migration in concentrated suspensions: Couette flow. *J. of Rheology* **35**: 773–797.

Assink, R. A., Caprihan, A., & Fukushima, E. 1989. Density profiles of a draining foam by nuclear magnetic resonance imaging. *AIChE J.* **34**: 2077–2081.

Callaghan, P. T. 1984. Pulsed field gradient nuclear magnetic resonance as a probe of liquid state molecular organization. *Australian J. Physics.* **37**: 359–387.

Callaghan, P. T., Jolley, K. W., & Humphrey, R. S. 1983. Diffusion of fat and water in cheese as studied by pulsed field gradient nuclear magnetic resonance. *J. Colloid and Interface Science* **93**: 521–529.

Callaghan, P. T., MacGowan, D., Packer, K. J., & Zelaya, F. O. 1990. High-resolution q-space imaging in porous structures. *J. Mag. Reson.* **90**: 177–182.

Carr, H. Y. & Purcell, E. M. 1954. Effects of diffusion on free precession in nuclear magnetic resonance experiments. *Physical Review* **94**: 630–638.

Cheng, W. C., Luthra, N. P., & Pereira, C. J. 1990. Study of restricted diffusion in porous catalysts by NMR. *AIChE J.* **36**: 559–568.

Cory, D. G., & Garroway, A. N. 1990. Measurement of translational displacement probabilities by NMR: An indicator of comparmentation. *Mag. Reson. in Med.* **14**: 435–444.

Hahn, E. L. 1950. Spin echoes. *Physical Review* **80**: 580–594.

Heil J. R., Özilgen, M., & McCarthy, M. J. 1993. Magnetic resonance imaging analysis of water migration and void formation in baking biscuits. *AIChE Symposium Series*, edited by G. Barbosa-Canosava and M. Okos, **297**: 39–45.

Kärger, J., Pfeifer, H., & Heink, W. 1988. Principles and applications of self-diffusion measurements by nuclear magnetic resonance. In *Advances in Magnetic Resonance*, edited by J. S. Waugh. New York: Academic Press.

Kauten, R. J., Maneval, J. E., & McCarthy, M. J. 1991. Fast determination of spatially localized volume fractions in emulsions. *J. of Food Science* **56**: 799–801, 847.

Klammler, F., & Kimmich, R. 1990. Volume-selective and spectroscopically resolved NMR investigation of diffusion and relaxation in fertilized hen eggs. *Physics in Medicine and Biology* **35**: 67–79.

Kose, K., 1990. NMR imaging of turbulent structure in a transitional pipe flow. *J. Phys. D: Appl. Phys.* **23**: 981–983.

Majors, P. D., Ackley, J. L., Altobelli, S. A., Caprihan, A., & Fukushima, E. 1990. Eddy current compensation by direct field detection and digital gradient modification. *J. Magn. Reson.* **87**: 548–553.

Maneval, J. E., McCarthy, M. J., & Whitaker, S. 1990. Use of nuclear magnetic resonance as an experimental probe in multiphase systems: Determination of the instrument weight function for measurements of liquid-phase volume fractions. *Water Resources Research* **26**: 2807–2816.

McCarthy, K. L., Kauten, R. J., & Agemura, C. K. 1992. Application of NMR imaging to the study of velocity profiles during extrusion processing. *Trends Fd Sci. and Tech.* **3**: 215–219.

McCarthy, K. L., Kauten, R. J., McCarthy, M. J., & Steffe, J. F. 1991. Flow profiles in a tube rheometer using magnetic resonance imaging. *J. of Food Engineering* **16**: 1–17.

McCarthy, M. J. 1990. Interpretation of the magnetic resonance imaging signal from a foam. *AIChE J.* **36**: 287–290.

McCarthy, M. J., Maneval, J., & Powell, R. L. 1992. Structure/property measurements using magnetic resonance spectroscopy and imaging. In *Advances in Food Engineering*, edited by R. P. Singh and A. Wirakartakamasuma. Boca Raton, FL: CRC Press.

Packer, K. J., & Rees, C. 1972. Pulsed NMR studies of restricted diffusion. I. Droplet size distributions in emulsions. *J. Colloidal and Interface Science.* **40**: 206–218.

Packer, K. J., & Zelaya, F. O. 1989. Observation of diffusion of fluids in porous solids by pulsed field gradient NMR. *Colloids and Surfaces* **36**: 221–227.

Philhofer, G. Master Thesis, University of California, Davis 1992.

Powell, R. L., Seymour, J., McCarthy, M. J., & McCarthy, K. 1992. Magnetic resonance imaging as a tool for rheological investigation. In *Theoretical and Applied Rheology:*

Proceedings of the XIth International Congress on Rheology, edited by Paula Moldenaers and Roland Keunings, 946–948. Amsterdam: Elsevier Science Publishers.

Sinton, S. W., & Chow, A. W. 1991. NMR flow imaging of fluids and solid suspensions in poiseuille flow, *J. Rheology* **35**: 735–772.

Stejskal, E. O. 1965. Use of spin echoes in a pulsed magnetic-field gradient to study anisotropic, restricted diffusion and flow. *J. of Chemical Physics.* **42**: 288–292.

Stejskal, E. O., & Tanner, J. E. 1965. Spin diffusion measurements: Spin echoes in the presence of a time-dependent field gradient. *J. Chemical Physics.* **43**: 3597–3603.

Stilbs, P. 1987. Fourier transform pulsed-field gradient spin echo studies of molecular diffusion. *Progress in NMR Spectroscopy* **19**: 1–45.

Tanner, J. E., & Stejskal, E. O. 1968. Restricted self-diffusion of protons in colloidal systems by the pulsed-gradient spin-echo method. *J. of Chemical Physics.* **49**: 1768–1777.

Taylor, D. G., & Bushell, M. C. 1985. The spatial mapping of translational diffusion coefficients by the NMR imaging technique. *Physics in Medicine and Biology.* **30**: 345–349.

Turney, M. 1990. Masters Thesis Department of Chemical Engineering, University of California, Davis.

Xia, Y., & Callaghan, P. T. 1990. The measurement of diffusion and flow of polymer solutions using dynamic NMR microscopy. *Makromolecular Chemie Macromolecular Symposium* **34**: 277–286.

4

Moisture and Lipid Distributions

Noninvasive measurement of moisture and lipid saturation distribution in foods is useful for improving product quality, product development, and processing. Magnetic resonance is well suited to the measurement of fat and moisture because these components generally have adequate concentrations for good signal-to-noise ratios and contributions from each component in the NMR signal can usually be separated in a straightforward manner (Winkler, McCarthy & German 1991).

Saturation Measurements

The following comments are directed primarily toward the measurement of saturations based on either spin-warp imaging, simple chemical shift imaging, or relaxation weighted imaging. Correct analysis of the transport of a particular component in a food or food system is possible only when there is correct information on saturation distribution, material structure, material properties, and thermodynamic data for the entire system. MRI can provide information on all of these items. However, given the limitations associated with MRI (for example, the technique does not directly relate to the enthalpy of an object), care must be exercised in designing experiments and interpreting the data. MRI should be considered a complementary, experimental technique to existing experimental methods.

Experimental Setup

Probe

Considerations regarding the electronics of the probe have been covered in Chapter 3, but the issue of the signal-to-noise (S/N) ratio will be covered here.

Many authors have discussed ways to optimize the S/N ratio and how the S/N ratio influences the quality of the image (Morris 1986; Mansfield & Morris 1982). However, in the case of food systems, it frequently happens that a signal from the object is strong enough to "saturate" the receiver, i.e., the signal is no longer accurately recorded and the response recorded by the ADC is a constant voltage. Whenever this occurs, the author has found it useful to include an attenuator in front of the receiver. Another way to deal with this situation is to replace the receiver with one that has a lower total amount of amplification. The advantage in MRI of studying samples with intrinsically good S/N ratios is that it is possible to use a probe that is large relative to sample size. This makes it possible to run several samples at a time and effectively minimizes variations in the B_1 field and probe response across the sample. For most of the birdcage coils that have been constructed in the author's laboratory, the region in the center of the coil has very good B_1 homogeneity and, consequently, a very linear response. Hence, the requirements for the B_1 field and general aspects of the probe design often do not need to be as stringent as in other types of studies (for example, high-resolution or solid-state NMR).

Other important factors concerning S/N ratio include imaging time, relaxation times, volume element size, and frequency of the spectrometer. Morris (1986) has detailed this relationship for cubic volume and a slice as follows:

$$t_{cubic\ volume} \cong \left(\frac{S}{N}\right)^{1/2} a^2 \left(\frac{T_1}{T_2}\right) \frac{1.418*10^{-15}}{v^{\frac{7}{2}} C} \left(\frac{1}{\Delta x}\right)^6 \qquad [4.1]$$

$$t_{slice} \cong \left(\frac{S}{N}\right)^{1/2} a^2 \left(\frac{T_1}{T_2}\right) \frac{1.418*10^{-15}}{v^{\frac{7}{2}} C} \left(\frac{1}{\Delta z}\right)^2 \left(\frac{1}{\Delta x}\right)^4 \qquad [4.2]$$

where $\boldsymbol{C}$ is a constant that depends on the flip angle and repetition rate (optimum value is 1/2), $\boldsymbol{a}$ is the receiver coil radius, and $\boldsymbol{v}$ is the resonance frequency in MHz. Note the dependence of imaging time, $\boldsymbol{t}$, on the 6th power of $\boldsymbol{\Delta x}$ for a cubic volume. As one attempts to achieve greater spatial resolution, the time required to keep a constant S/N ratio increases rapidly.

Sample Container

For measurement of component saturations, it is advantageous to minimize susceptibility variations related to sample geometry whenever possible. The shape of the sample is important just as it is in high-resolution NMR studies. In order to minimize susceptibility variations, the best shapes for samples are spherical, cylindrical, or toroidal (doughnut-shaped). Susceptibility variations induced by the geometry of the sample are eliminated only when the sample is an infinite cylinder or a perfect toroid or a perfect sphere. However, it is frequently not possible to attain geometries that minimize geometry-induced susceptibility variations because of construction constraints for simulated process equipment or because there is an even greater need to simplify the mathematical analysis of the phenomena. The material of choice for many sample containers is plastic. It can be easily machined and fabricated into complex geometries. If many similar types of samples are to be analyzed, it is often helpful to build a positioning device within the electronic probe. Students in the author's laboratory have utilized everything from Styrofoam® (Dow Chemical Co.) to cardboard as temporary positioning devices. More permanent holders are made of plastic and the probe is dovetailed for highly accurate placement (Fig. 4.1).

Spectrometer Setup

As discussed in Chapter 3, precautions need to be taken to ensure that the spectrometer is set up properly. Additionally, when doing chemical shift imaging, great care should be taken to homogenize the field. Just as in high-resolution NMR, if the shimming is poor the results are difficult to interpret.

Analysis of the NMR Signal

Spin-Warp Imaging

The signal strength in each voxel is given by:

$$S(\mathbf{r}) = K(\mathbf{r})\exp(-TE/T_2(\mathbf{r}))(1-\exp(-TR/T_1(\mathbf{r})) \qquad [4.3]$$

where the constant, ***K***, includes the number density of the nuclei and the constants related to hardware, ***TE*** is echo time, and ***TR*** is the predelay. It is important to recognize that, in general, the signal strength, constant of proportionality, nuclei density, and relaxation times will all vary with position within the sample. Thus, the most general case for determination of concentrations requires the analysis of how relaxation times vary and how the response of the system (K(**r**)) varies.

Relaxation Effects

The signal strength depends exponentially on the relaxation times. Consequently, small changes in the relaxation times produce significant variations in signal strength (see Table 4.1). The calculation in Table 4.1 assumes a single value for the spin spin relaxation time. If this is the case, only two acquisitions at different TE values (in principle) are needed to calculate the T_2 value at each position. Using the equation:

$$T_2 = (TE_1 - TE_2)/\log(S_2/S_1) \qquad [4.4]$$

the T_2 can be estimated and the signal corrected by the following:

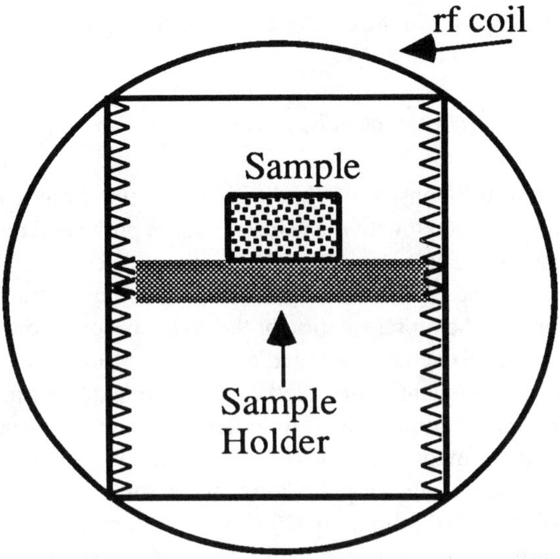

Figure 4.1. Example of a probe configuration for precise sample placement.

Table 4.1. Variation of signal strength with spin spin relaxation time (TE = 20 ms, TR>>5T_1).

$\exp(-TE/T_2)$	T_2 (ms)
0.9802	1000
0.9608	500
0.8187	100
0.6703	50
0.5134	30
0.4493	25
0.3679	20
0.2636	15
0.1353	10

$$S = \frac{S_1}{\exp(-TE_1/T_2)} \qquad [4.5]$$

where S is the corrected signal strength, subs 1 and 2 refer to acquisitions 1 and 2 at different TE (McCarthy 1990).

When the relaxation is not exponential, multiple relaxation times are used to fit the decay of the signal. For the case of two transverse relaxation time constants, the signal is given by ($TR >> T_1$):

$$S(\mathbf{r}) = K'(\mathbf{r})[\phi_a(\mathbf{r})\exp(-TE/T_{2a}(\mathbf{r})) + \phi_b(\mathbf{r})\exp(-TE/T_{2b}(\mathbf{r}))] \qquad [4.6]$$

where ϕ is the number density of spin with a specific T_2 and $K'(\mathbf{r})$ describes only the constants associated with the response of the probe and receiver network. The representation of the signal becomes more complicated if T_1 weighting occurs or if more than two time constants are needed to describe the transverse decay of the magnetization. As the representation of the signal becomes more complicated, more data is required to achieve a reliable estimate of the relaxation times and percentages of the components associated with each relaxation time constant. The experimental time and computational time needed to achieve spatially resolved component saturation maps and relaxation time maps can be significant. For example, if a standard spin-warp imaging pulse sequence is used to acquire twenty points for a T_2 determination, 20 times the normal experimental time is needed. Also, significant data processing is required to estimate all parameters. This method of estimating variations in relaxation times may fail if conditions in the sample change before the complete data set can be acquired. An approach used with some success is to approximate a multi-exponential decay as a single exponential decay and accept the additional error introduced. Clearly the adequacy of this technique depends on the experimental settings and sample relaxation times as shown in Table 4.2.

Temperature Effects

The NMR signal is proportional to ($1/T_a$) where T_a is the absolute temperature. In the majority of experiments, temperature variations across a sample should not have a measurable effect on the signal intensity. However, if large gradients exist, temperature-induced variations in signal intensity can occur. Processes in which this might be observed are microwave heating and immersion freezing.

Quantification of Water and Lipid Signals

Two general approaches exist to separate and quantify the spatial distribution of water and lipid components: relaxation weighted techniques and chemical shift imaging. Relaxation-weighted techniques are well suited to quantifying the spatial distribution of water and lipid. However, measurements of actual component concentrations with relaxation-weighted imaging is not a simple procedure. On the other hand, chemical shift imaging can provide the component concentrations and spatial distributions in one experiment, but a chemical shift imaging experiment requires significantly more time than a relaxation-weighted image.

Table 4.2. Error associated with ignoring multiexponential decays for signal correction.

Phase Vol. A	TE_1 (ms)	TE_2 (ms)	T_{2a} (ms)	T_{2b} (ms)	Error %
0.5	10	30	10	100	15
0.5	10	30	50	100	0
0.5	10	20	50	500	1
0.1	10	20	10	100	3
0.1	10	20	50	100	0
0.1	10	20	50	500	0
0.5	15	20	10	100	14
0.5	15	20	50	100	0
0.5	15	20	50	500	1
0.1	15	20	10	100	4
0.1	15	20	100	500	0
0.1	15	20	50	800	0
0.1	15	30	10	500	6
0.1	15	20	250	500	0
0.1	15	30	30	200	1

The first requirement for relaxation-weighted imaging is that the water and lipid have either different T_1 or T_2 time constants. In order to produce satisfactory contrast (enhancement of signal from one component relative to another), the relaxation times should be different by at least a factor of 2. Figure 4.2 shows the signal ratio between two components of equal saturation as a function of the difference in T_1 relaxation times and predelay settings. Figure 4.3 demonstrates the contrast available from spin spin relaxation time differences using conditions similar to those illustrated in Figure 4.2. The most important conclusion from these plots is that it is generally not possible to totally separate the signal from two different components based solely on relaxation times.

In order to quantify component concentrations, the best approach is to use chemical shift imaging or localized spectroscopy. A chemical shift image experiment can generate a two-, three-, or four-dimensional data set for each time step. Analysis of component concentrations proceeds in the same manner as for high-resolution spectroscopy. The resonance line shapes are fit with a Lorentzian function and the areas then compared to a standard calibration. Although this procedure is time-consuming, it provides a generally accurate measure of nuclei density per volume. Conversion of this numerical value to normal concentration units is discussed in the next section.

Relationship of Signal Intensities to Concentration Values

For most engineering and quality assurance applications, the standard units for a concentration (for moisture) are grams of component per gram of dry solids.

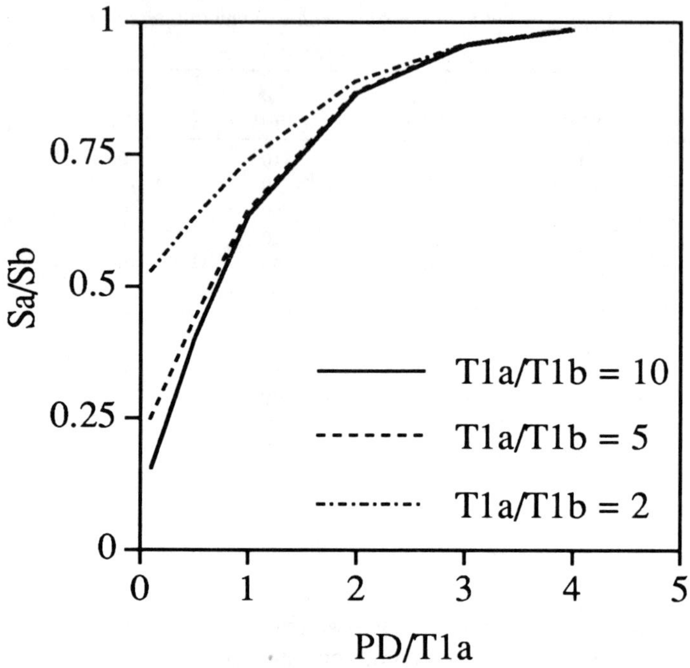

Figure 4.2. Ratio of signal intensities from two components ***a*** and ***b*** as a function of predelay time divided by T_1 of component ***a***.

Almost all literature uses this or an equivalent set of units. In MRI measurements of concentration, the units for the data are quantity of nuclei per unit volume. The issue then is how to perform the conversion of MRI data to standard form and what unit volume to use.

Conversion between MRI data in grams/volume to grams/gram dry solids is trivial if the solid matrix is constant and uniform. Then it is necessary to measure only a single standard and ratio the signal intensity to the standard in order to obtain an accurate conversion. For example:

$$\text{Standard: } \frac{g/g \text{ dry solids}}{\text{signal/unit volume}}$$

$$\text{Signal: } \frac{\text{signal}}{\text{unit volume}}$$

The conversion becomes difficult, however, when the material being studied shrinks or expands or when the solid matrix is nonhomogeneous. The conversion becomes a case-by-case procedure when variations in solids distribution occurs. There are several approaches which can generally achieve acceptable results. One method is to ignore slight changes and assume that the solid matrix is

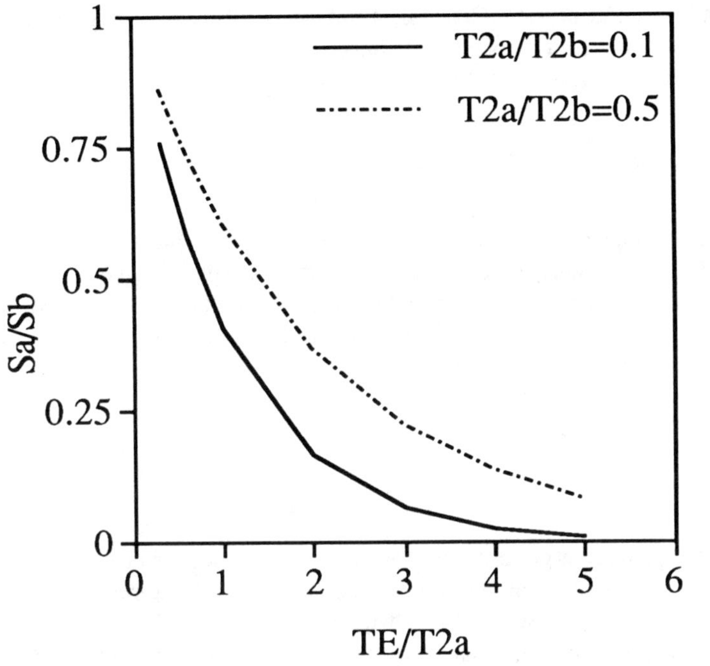

Figure 4.3. Relative signal intensity of component ***a*** to component ***b*** in a spin echo experiment for different ratios of T_2.

essentially uniform. This procedure has been used with success in the drying of apples and potatoes (McCarthy, Perez & Özilgen 1991; Ruan et al. 1991). When there are changes in volume or when the inherent distribution is significantly nonuniform, a mathematical description of the solids distribution is needed; in the most general case, this is a function of time and space.

Consider, for example, the case of drying a cellular material. The goal is to determine two quantities: the spatial average density of nonaqueous material and the mass average velocity, **W*** (Crapiste, Whitaker & Rotstein 1988). Assuming unidirectional shrinkage and that shrinkage is a function of water content only, it can be shown that the shrinkage is given by:

$$L_o^n = n\int_0^{L(t)} (\xi^{n-1}/S^*)d\xi \qquad [4.7]$$

and

$$\mathbf{W}^* = -\frac{S^*}{\xi^{n-1}}\int_0^{\xi} [\chi^{n-1}\frac{d(1/S^*)}{dx^*}\frac{\partial x^*}{\partial t}]d\chi \qquad [4.8]$$

with $\mathbf{W}^* = 0$ at $\xi = 0$ (Crapiste, Whitaker & Rotstein 1988). Conversion of MRI saturation data into normal units will need to utilize equations such as Equations 4.7 and 4.8.

Moisture Saturation Measurements

Moisture saturation measurements are probably the most extensively applied measurements in nonmedical MRI. Most of these studies have centered on measuring the moisture saturation and the variation in relaxation times with moisture content and temperature. The materials studied fall into two broad categories: agricultural products and porous media.

Drying of Agricultural Products

Apples

Apples provide a good model system to study moisture migration in cellular materials. They are relatively homogeneous, have a high moisture content, and have relaxation times which make MRI relatively easy. Studies of apple drying have determined the changes in spin spin relaxation time and spin lattice relaxation time with moisture content (Perez, Kauten & McCarthy 1988). In a subsequent study, moisture profiles during the initial stages of drying were used to determine effective moisture diffusivities (McCarthy, Perez & Özilgen 1991). Since shrinkage was negligible during the early stage of drying, MRI data was directly converted to standard moisture concentration of g water/g dry solids. Figure 4.4 shows the changing moisture profiles in an apple slab during drying. This figure demonstrates the slight error of assuming a uniform moisture content in the apple and hence a universal conversion factor.

Potatoes

Another model study of drying determined effective moisture diffusivities during dehydration and rehydration in potato tissue (Ruan et al. 1991). Similar to the apple drying work, average moisture contents were used to scale (or convert) the MRI signals into standard units. In addition, limited moisture content ranges were analyzed for calculating effective diffusivities (40–55% wet basis for dehydration and 56–60% for absorption). The additional challenge in this study was the actual heating of the sample to typical drying temperatures. The transverse and longitudinal relaxation times were shown to vary with temperature. Ruan and co-workers chose to vary the TE during the experiment in order to maintain a constant ratio of TE/T_2. This was done in order to simplify data analysis so that during the entire experiment only one constant (or standard value)

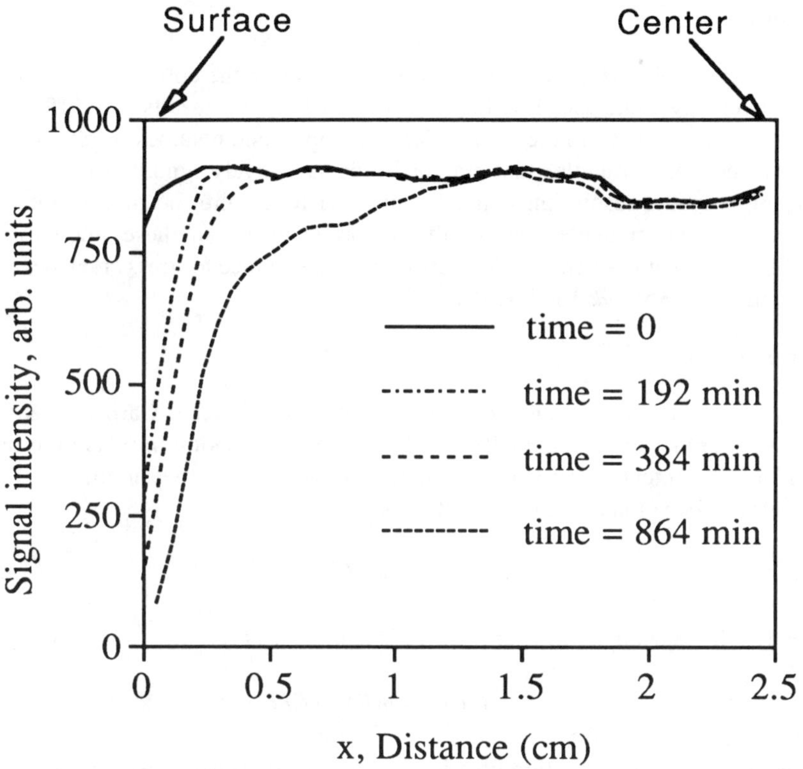

Figure 4.4. Moisture profiles in an apple slab during air drying. Signal intensity is proportional to moisture content.

was needed to convert MRI signals to moisture saturations as shown in the expression:

$$f = K \exp(-TE/T_2) \qquad [4.9]$$

where f is the constant of proportionality between moisture content and signal intensity.

While this approach used by Ruan was successful for one study, great care must be taken when applying the technique to other experiments (Ruan et al. 1991). For this approach to be accurate, the relaxation times of the sample cannot depend on position and, additionally, temperature gradients within the sample should be small. Otherwise the relaxation times vary spatially and each voxel can be weighted by a different $\exp(-TE/T_2)$ value. This type of spatial weighting of relaxation rate, if it occurs, renders the technique unreliable.

Corn

The drying of corn (both individual kernels and on the cob) has been studied extensively by Song and Litchfield (1989, 1990). The results are different in two major respects from the studies done on apples and potatoes. First, corn has a heterogeneous structure that cannot be presumptively ignored and, second, very high spatial resolution is needed in order to acquire meaningful moisture saturation measurements. One of the important results of these studies is the confirmation that gradients in moisture content are related to stress crack development in corn (Song & Litchfield 1990).

Drying of Gels

Moisture content measurements in gels demonstrate (Duce, Carpenter & Hall 1990b; Schrader & Litchfield 1992) how to use the variation in relaxation times with solids content to convert MRI data to concentration measurements. If the predelay between acquisitions is set to $5T_1$:

$$S = K\rho\exp(-TE/T_2) \qquad [4.10]$$

This can be rearranged to (Schrader & Litchfield 1992):

$$Ln(S/\rho) = Ln(K) - TE/T_2 \qquad [4.11]$$

Since the spin spin relaxation time in many gel systems is inversely proportional to concentration, the equation becomes:

$$C = \frac{1}{K'TE}[Ln(K) - Ln(S/\rho)] \qquad [4.12]$$

where K' is the constant of proportionality between $1/T_2$ and concentration of solids in the gel, and C is the concentration of solids in the unknown. If proton density changes only slightly with solids concentration, the ln(S) becomes proportional to concentration (Schrader & Litchfield 1992).

Drying of Porous Media

Use of Zero-, One-, and Two-dimensional Data

MRI data should be acquired only when necessary since the technique is both expensive and time-consuming. Drying of a porous media is a system that illustrates the utility of data with zero-, one-, or two-dimensional spatial information (as shown in Figure 4.5). Zero-dimensional data is acquired without any spatial encoding of the signal and is a bulk measurement of the moisture content.

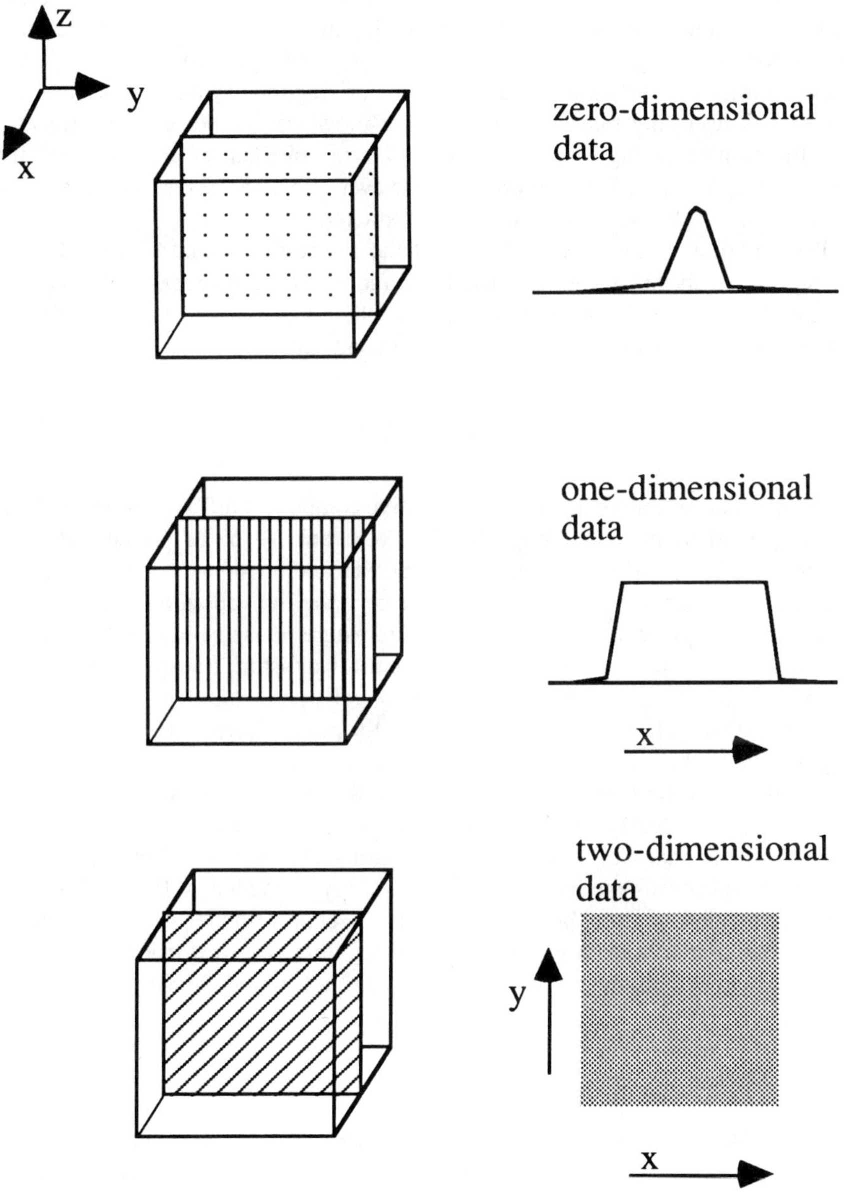

Figure 4.5. Illustration of the different types of spatially resolved signal available from a plane selected in a three-dimensional object.

A one-dimensional set of data is the signal integrated over a plane perpendicular to the direction of interest. A two-dimensional data set is a set of density values within one plane, with each intensity value having a separate value of the other two coordinates (e.g., $\rho(x_1, y_1, z_1)$, $r(x_1, y_2, z_1)$, $r(x_1, y_3, z_1)$).

Zero-dimensional data is useful for characterizing the drying rate curve of the material. The drying rate curve is a plot of moisture lost per unit surface area as a function of drying time (Figure 4.6). Drying rate curves are useful for the engineering design of a drying process; however, the plot does not provide much information on the physics of the drying process.

The addition of spatial distribution of the moisture content allows effective moisture diffusivities to be calculated and more advanced theories of drying to be tested (Crapiste, Whitaker & Rotstein 1988). Effective moisture diffusivities can be calculated from the use of Fick's second law (in 1-D):

$$\frac{\partial^2 C}{\partial t} = D\frac{\partial^2 C}{\partial x^2} \qquad [4.13]$$

where C is concentration and D is the effective component diffusivity. Procedures can be found in the monograph by Crank (Crank 1975) to predict effective diffusivities for a variety of different geometries and boundary conditions. More advanced theories of moisture transport incorporate the structure of the material into the model (for example, the theory of moisture transport in cellular systems by Crapiste and co-workers, 1988). A model for moisture transport through the cell wall and through air spaces between the cells predicted drying rates during the initial stages; after the structure changed, the model failed (Crapiste, Whitaker & Rotstein 1988).

Details about the structure and changes in the structure can be obtained with two-dimensional MRI data. Maneval and co-workers have demonstrated the use of two-dimensional data to characterize length scales that are of importance for the drying of porous media (Maneval, McCarthy & Whitaker 1990). The two-dimensional information helped to validate a simple model of mass transfer during the first falling rate period. However, this two-dimensional data was inadequate to explain the physics of the constant rate period (Maneval, McCarthy & Whitaker 1990).

Film Thickness Measurements

The displacement of a spin is an effective method to measure the droplet size distribution in an emulsion (as previously discussed in Chapter 3). The same procedure can be used to measure the permeability of a membrane and the thickness of a liquid film on a surface. Determining if a liquid film exists on a surface and measuring the thickness of the film should help to improve the description of the mechanisms responsible for moisture transport during drying.

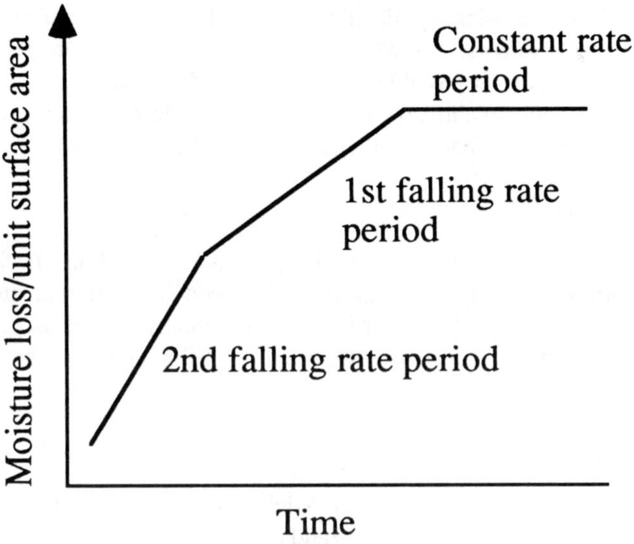

Figure 4.6. Idealized drying rate curve.

In the extension of pulsed field gradient studies to measuring film thickness, the influence of the evaporation-condensation process at the air-water interface must be considered. There are two limiting factors that are relevant when doing NMR studies. The first case occurs when the rate of evaporation is slow compared to the diffusion within the film. In this case, the gas-liquid interface behaves simply as a solid-liquid interface and a no-flux condition can be used for this boundary. The second case occurs when spin transport is rapid at the gas-liquid interface with respect to diffusion in the liquid film. In this instance, at longer echo times, films with a larger surface area have a significantly reduced signal intensity. The result is a measurement that primarily reflects only the structure of the area of liquid with a small surface area. Confirmation that this process is actually occurring can be made if the gain required to observe the signals is attenuated to a greater extent than the decrease in moisture saturation.

Pulsed field gradient studies of a glass bead-air-water system were made by Maneval (1991). Film thicknesses of 20–30 μm were measured and found to be almost independent of saturation. This indicates that even at low saturations, water exists in a state similar to that at high saturations. The results of this study are consistent with the models currently proposed to explain the constant rate period of drying (Schlünder 1988; Suzuki & Maeda 1968).

Lipid Saturation Measurements

An excellent discussion of the state-of-the-art MRI methods to separate water and fat signals has been written by Kaldoudi and Williams (1992). Although this article addresses medical applications, the methods are in most cases directly applicable to food systems. The MRI techniques used to separate fat and water signals are based on the different NMR properties of fat and water, for example, relaxation time, chemical shift, or scalar coupling (Kaldoudi & Williams 1992). There is no single pulse sequence that is successful in all systems.

Medical

Differentiation of water and fat signals is important for studying fat infiltration of the liver and heart or for distinguishing between two different tumor types (Kaldoudi & Williams 1992; Morris 1986). Additionally, noninvasive measurements of body fat are important in studying the development and changes in the body.

Animal

NMR is useful in studying live animals. MRI is currently being used to measure water/fat distribution, muscle structure, and the influence of different feed formulations on the animal (Beauvallet & Renou 1992). Measurement of water and fat content can be performed on live animals or on carcasses. In addition to measures of saturation, the detailed distribution of fat in the animal or in a specific organ is possible. Renou has recently demonstrated that lipids in each lobe of a goose liver have different globule sizes (Beauvallet & Renou 1992). MRI in combination with other NMR techniques are proving useful in evaluation of animal feeding and breeding experiments.

Processed Food

One of the most important issues for processed food quality is preventing moisture and lipid components from migrating to different regions of a food product, for example, the diffusion of water from a cookie filling into the baked shell. MRI is probably the best technique for noninvasively following the diffusion of lipid and water in foods (McCarthy & Kauten 1990). This was demonstrated by following the movement of fat into bread from a natural peanut butter filling. The MRI signal was relaxation weighted to show primarily the lipid component and hence fat diffusion into the bread.

Overall very few processed foods have had their water and lipid content measured with MRI. Most of the studies are on simulated foods or model systems. Duce and co-workers (Duce, Carpenter & Hall 1990a) have used MRI to look at the lipid crystallization in chocolate and this will be discussed in the next chapter. Heil, Özilgen, and McCarthy (1992) used localized spectroscopy and MRI to study the void formation, lipid migration, and moisture loss in American-style biscuits during and after baking. The results were similar to the data previously reported in the literature showing an increase in moisture content in the center of the biscuit immediately after baking and little, if any, lipid migration. Heil has also demonstrated a simple NMR procedure for quantifying the amount of oil in dressings (Heil, Perkins & McCarthy 1990). The procedure relies solely on knowledge of the container geometry and that the oil and water phases will be separated. As shown in Chapter 1, Figure 1.17 is a one-dimensional profile of oil and water in a container with a spike at the interface due to a chemical shift artifact. Hence the phase volumes can be calculated from this type of one-dimensional image. The potential exists to use MRI to study a variety of phenomena important to processed food quality, for example, lipid and moisture distribution in frozen foods, shelf-stable foods, microwaved meals, and fried foods. Figure 4.7 illustrates the difficulty in data analysis for these types of systems. Figure 4.7 shows just the contour plots of hydrogen density in a potato before

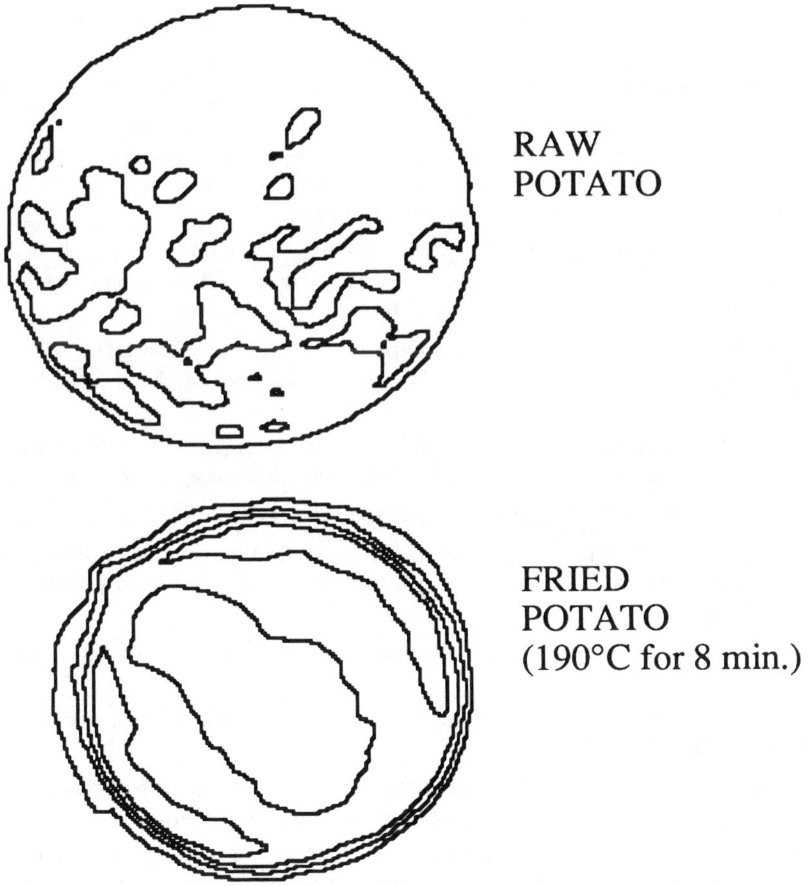

Figure 4.7. Contour plots of hydrogen density in raw and fried potato.

and after frying. Note the shrinkage and the dramatic change in signal variations. Analysis of frying using MRI is just beginning and has been limited to semiquantitative analysis (Farkas, Singh & McCarthy 1992).

References

Beauvallet, C., & Renou, J-P. 1992. Applications of NMR spectroscopy in meat research. *Trends in Food Science and Technology* **3**: 241–246.

Crank, J. 1975. *The Mathematics of Diffusion*. New York: Oxford University Press.

Crapiste, G. H., Whitaker, S., & Rotstein, E. 1988. Drying of cellular material I. A mass transfer theory. *Chem. Engr. Sci.* **43**: 2919–2928.

Duce, S. L., Carpenter, T. A., & Hall, L. D. 1990a. Nuclear magnetic resonance imaging of chocolate confectionery and the spatial detection of polymorphic states of cocoa butter in chocolate. *Lebensmittel-Wissenschaft und-Technologie* **23**: 565–569.

Duce, S. L., Carpenter, T. A., & Hall, L. D. 1990b. Use of n.m.r. imaging to map the spatial distrubution [*sic*] of structure in polysaccharide gels. *Carbohydrate Research* C1-C4.

Farkas, B. E., Singh, R. P., & McCarthy, M. J. 1992. Measurement of oil/water interface in foods during frying. In *Advances in Food Engineering,* edited by R. P. Singh and A. Wirakartakamasuma. Boca Raton, FL:CRC Press.

Heil, J. R., Özilgen, M. & McCarthy, M. J. 1993. Magnetic resonance imaging analysis of water migration and void formation in baking biscuits. *AIChE Symposium* Series, edited by G. Barbosa-Canosava and M. Okos, **297**: 39–45.

Heil, J. R., Perkins, W. E., & McCarthy, M. J. 1990. Use of magnetic resonance procedures for measurement of oil in French style dressings. *J. Food Sci.* **55**: 763–764.

Kaldoudi, E., & Williams, S. R. C. 1992. Fat and water differentiation by nuclear magnetic resonance imaging. *Concepts in Magnetic Resonance* **4**: 53–72, 162–165.

Maneval, J. E. 1991. Ph.D. University of California, Davis.

Maneval, J. E., McCarthy, M. J. and Whitaker, S. 1990 (August). Studies of the drying process by NMR imaging. *Proceedings of the 7th International Drying Symposium*, Prague, Czechoslovakia.

Mansfield, P., & Morris, P. G. 1982. *NMR Imaging in Biomedicine*. New York: Academic Press.

McCarthy, M. J. 1990. Interpretation of the magnetic resonance imaging signal from a foam. *AIChE J.* **36**: 287–290.

McCarthy, M. J., & Kauten, R. J. 1990. Magnetic resonance imaging applications in food research. *Trends in Food Science and Technology* **1**: 134–139.

McCarthy, M. J., Perez, E., & Özilgen, M. 1991. Model for transient moisture profiles of a drying apple slab using the data obtained with magnetic resonance imaging. *Biotechnology Progress* **7**: 540–543.

Morris, P. G. 1986. *Nuclear Magnetic Resonance Imaging in Medicine and Biology*. New York: Oxford University Press.

Perez, E., Kauten, R., & McCarthy, M. J. 1988 (August). Noninvasive measurement of moisture profiles during the drying of an apple. *Proceedings of the 6th International Drying Symposium*, Versailles, France.

Ruan, R., Schmidt, S. J., Schmidt, A. R., & Litchfield, J. B. 1991. Nondestructive measurement of transient moisture profiles and the moisture diffusion coefficient in a potato during drying and absorption by NMR imaging. *J. of Food Process Engineering* **14**: 297–313.

Schlünder, E.-U. 1988. On the mechanism of the constant drying-rate period and its relevance to diffusion-controlled catalytic gas-phase reactions. *Chem. Eng. Sci.* **43**: 2685–2689.

Schrader, G. W., & Litchfield, J. B. 1992. Moisture profiles in a model food gel during drying measurement using magnetic resonance imaging and evaluation of the Fickian model. *Drying Technology* **10**: 295–332.

Song, H., & Litchfield, J. B. 1989. Nondestructive measurement of transient, 3-D moisture transfer in corn during drying using NMR imaging. *Proceedings American Society of Agricultural Engineers*. New Orleans, Louisiana.

Song, H., & Litchfield, J. B. 1990. Nuclear magnetic resonance imaging of transient three-dimensional moisture distribution in an ear of corn during drying. *Cereal Chemistry* **67**: 580–584.

Suzuki, M., & Maeda, S. 1968. On the mechanism of drying granular beds. J. *Chem. Engr. Japan* **1**: 26–31.

Winkler, M. M., McCarthy, M. J., & German, J. B. 1991. Noninvasive measurement of lipid and water in food using magnetic resonance imaging. *J. Food Sci.* **56**: 811–815.

5

Phase Transitions

The texture and structure of many foods are either controlled or influenced by the liquid-solid phase transitions of water and/or lipids. A liquid-solid phase transition is traditionally studied using either calorimetry or low-resolution NMR. Both of these experimental approaches average the information obtained from a sample over the entire sample. Magnetic resonance imaging provides complementary information to the standard experimental approaches. MRI can be used to quantify the kinetics of phase transitions during simulated processing. This kinetic data is a stringent test of the current mathematical models of heat transfer and crystallization.

Quantification

Experimental Setup

Probe

A standard birdcage coil or temperature-controlled probe can be used to measure crystallization or melting. As in all other measurements of dynamic phenomena, care must be taken to ensure that the tuning of the probe does not change over the course of the experiment.

The author has had good results with placing the probe next to the surface of the freezing chamber and insulating over the probe. Under these circumstances, tuning becomes somewhat of a mechanical challenge; however, the benefit in stable probe temperatures and signal-to-noise ratio make it worth the small amount of time and effort required.

Sample Container

The heat transfer characteristics of the container and sample need careful consideration. For phase transitions within a container, the convective heat transfer from the surrounding media to the container wall and the conductive heat transfer through the container wall and into the sample need to be characterized. Measuring ice crystallization dynamics requires a temperature-controlled probe. Sometimes characterization of lipid crystallization can be performed using no temperature control; this procedure works well if the melting point is significantly above room temperature (Simoneau et al. 1991). Hence, the room air serves as the temperature control medium.

Process Equipment

Typical types of equipment that can be simulated include air-blast freezers, cryogenic freezers, and scraped-surface heat exchangers. Air-blast and cryogenic freezers can be inexpensively simulated in a batch mode. At the University of California, Davis, researchers have modified a pilot-scale air-blast freezer. The modifications replace the door of the freezer and add a divider in the freezing chamber (see Fig. 5.1). Several items that should be included in the modified door are a sensor to measure air flow rate and a thermocouple. Cryogenic freezers can be modified or simulated in a similar fashion.

The most challenging part of the design is often the sample handling section for rapid changing of the sample. In our air-blast freezing system, an end cap was added to the turn in the PVC pipe assembly as it exited the magnet and curved to recirculate the cold air, Fig. 5.2. The end cap could be removed easily and the sample was placed on a plastic sled with a long wooden handle. The sled moved on two small rails installed on the inside of the pipe. A stop was placed on the rails to make positioning reproducible from sample to sample.

A scraped-surface heat exchanger would be best simulated by building a simple analog for use in the spectrometer. The process to design and build the device would be the same as for the tube rheometer described in Chapter 3.

Another concern is for the audible noise that pilot-scale process equipment often makes. This noise can make the spectrometer room very uncomfortable and in some cases it may necessitate ear protection. Most of the devices the author has used have been either designed to have motors situated outside the spectrometer room or have been modified in such a manner shortly after the first use.

Spectrometer Setup

An additional factor to be considered in spectrometer setup/operation is the need to prevent interference from electrical noise generated by a compressor or fan motor. The author has not encountered serious noise problems with any motors. However, almost every piece of simulated process equipment required the installation of a new electrical circuit. During the installation, care was taken to isolate the motor from the spectrometer.

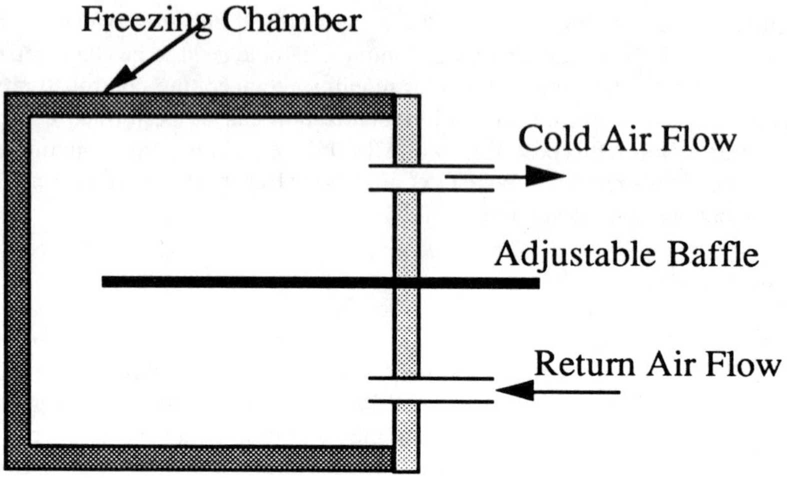

Figure 5.1. Modifications to a pilot-scale air-blast freezer for use with an MRI spectrometer.

Analysis of the NMR Signal

Relaxation Effects

MRI can be used to quantify the dynamics of crystallization and melting primarily because the signal depends on the relaxation times of the material. As a component crystallizes, the rate at which it returns to equilibrium in an NMR experiment changes dramatically. The spin spin relaxation rate can vary several orders of magnitude for typical food components between the liquid and the solid states. For example, consider the freezing of the beefsteak that is shown in Figure 5.3. The images are standard coronal spin-warp images of the beef in a simulated air-blast freezer. The dark circles are from thermocouples inserted into the samples. Note the bright edges near the thermocouples that are most likely susceptibility artifacts. If the images are acquired with a predelay >> T_1 of the solid or liquid phases, the water signal intensity is given by:

$$S_w = \rho_{ws}\exp(-TE/T_{2s}) + \rho_{wl}\exp(-TE/T_{2l}) \qquad [5.1]$$

where sub-*w* refers to water and sub-*l,s* refers to liquid or solid state. Since TE values are on the order of ms, while T_2 values for ice are on the order of μs, Equation 5.1 reduces to:

$$S_w = \rho_{wl}\exp(-TE/T_{2l}) \qquad [5.2]$$

Thus, the signal represents only the liquid phase. If all of the water begins the process in a liquid state, the decrease in signal intensity can be related directly

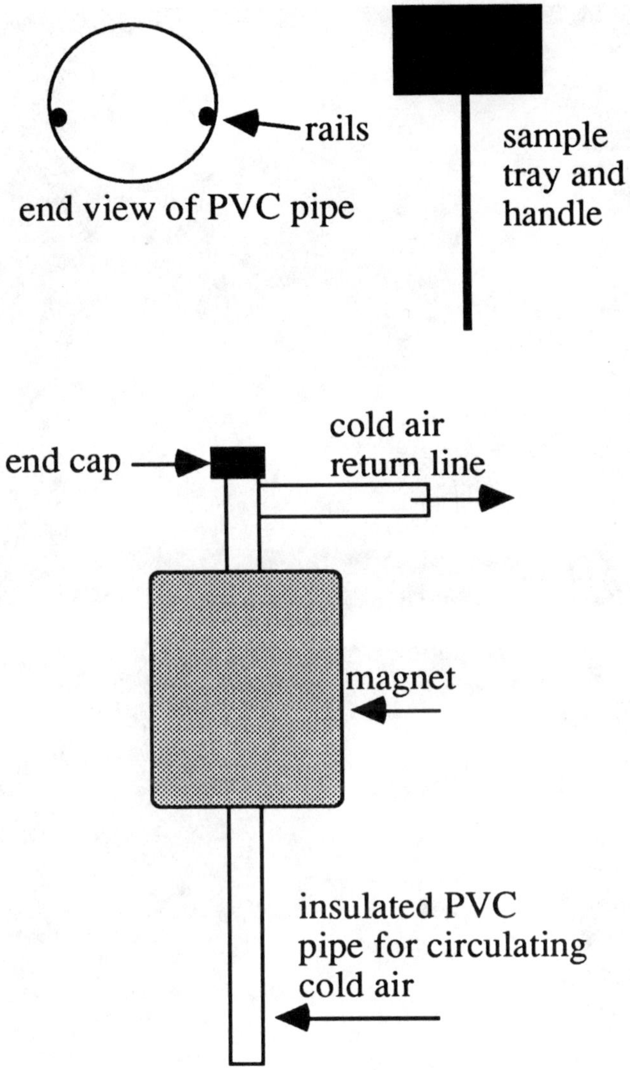

Figure 5.2. A simple system for changing the sample.

to a solid-liquid ratio at all times during the experiment, as long as temperature effects are not important.

Temperature Effects

A plot typical of the decrease in signal intensity is shown in Figure 5.4. The initial rise in signal is not always measurable. The initial rise is primarily due to the 1/Ta dependence of the NMR signal and is exaggerated on the plot for

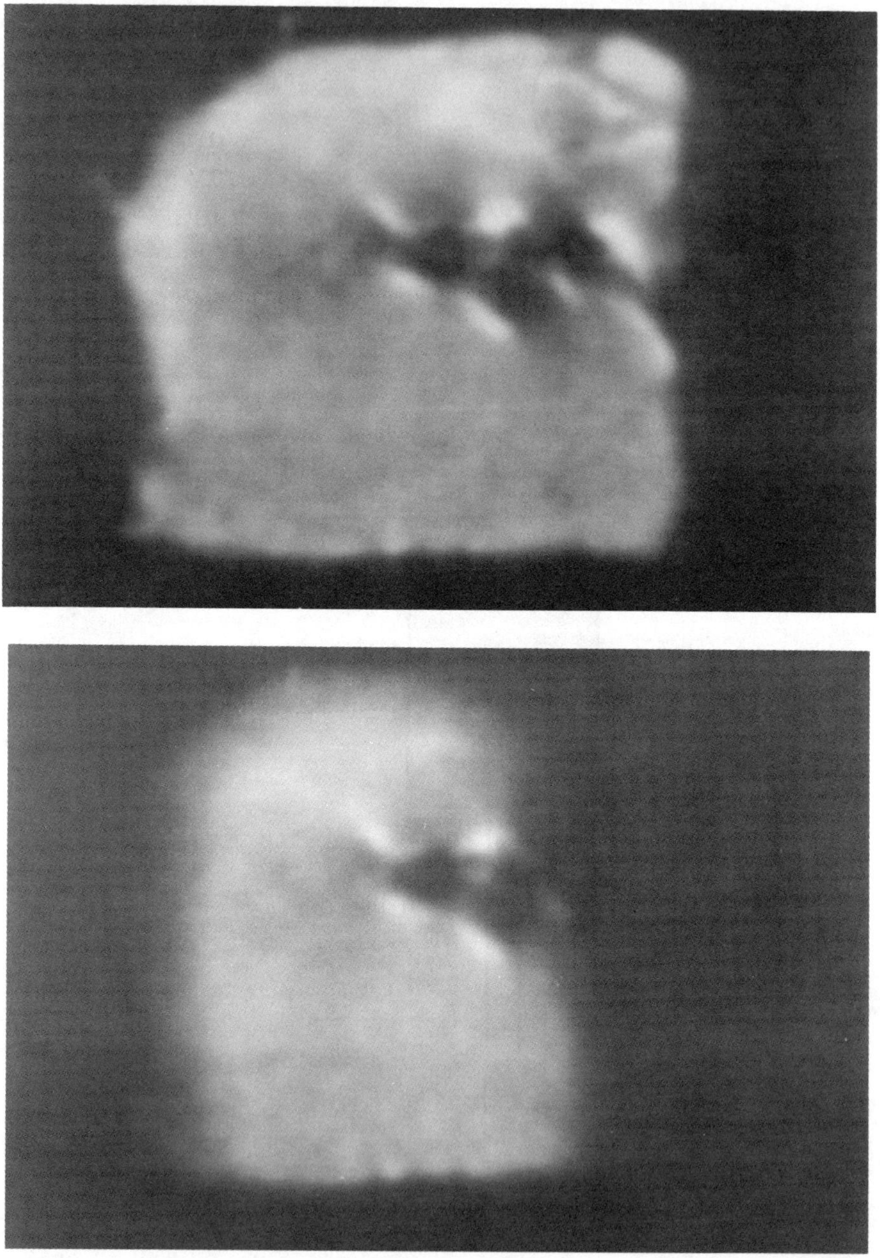

Figure 5.3. Freezing of a beefsteak in a simulated air-blast freezer. The top image was taken 3 minutes after placing the sample in the freezer, and the bottom image was taken 20 minutes after insertion.

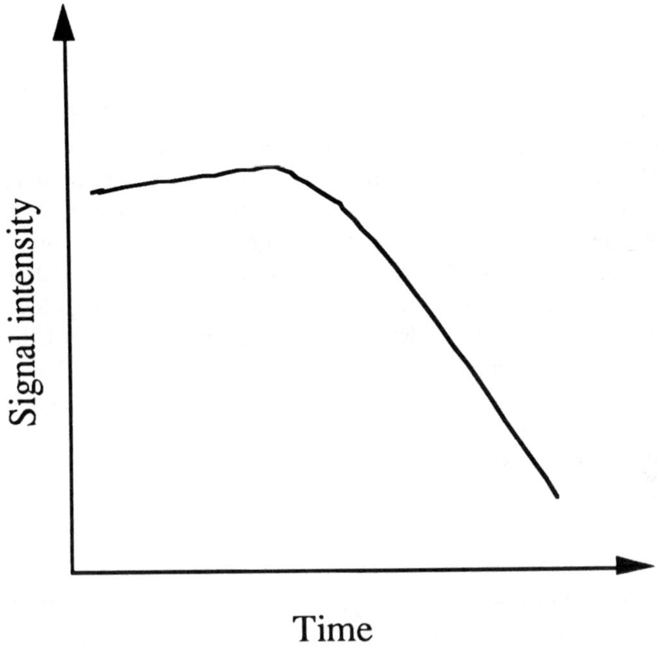

Figure 5.4. Change in NMR signal intensity as a liquid is cooled.

clarity. The temperature dependence follows Curie's law where the signal strength times the absolute temperature is a constant. It may be possible to generate regions of significant subcooling during the rapid freezing of food products. This subcooling may be great enough to result in a significant increase in signal intensity at the freezing interface which might influence the slope of the cooling curve shown in Figure 5.4. The author knows of no observations to this effect other than in a qualitative fashion during the freezing of irregular-shaped food products (McCarthy et al. 1991). However, as noted, other factors could have contributed to the observed changes in signal intensity, for example, geometric changes resulting in composition changes in a voxel.

When a significant portion of the water in the sample is frozen, the contribution from dissolved macromolecules needs to be accounted for (Harz, Weisser & Liebenspacher 1989). The method for correction of the freezing curve is to determine the solute concentration, C_f, the ratio of proton densities of solute to water, K, and use the following equation:

$$\varepsilon(\tau) = \phi(\tau)\cdot(K\cdot C_i + 1 - C_i)/(1 - C_i) \qquad [5.3]$$

where $\varepsilon(\tau)$ is the ratio of frozen water/initial water and C_i is the initial solute concentration.

Phase Volume Changes

When water and lipids are in a solid state their density decreases, and this results in an expansion of volume. For traditional low-resolution NMR measurements of crystallization, expansion does not need to be considered in the analysis. However, for MRI measurements, the change in density gives rise to small errors in measurement of crystallization dynamics. In the case of water, the error is probably insignificant. However, in the case of many lipids, the change in density can be as high as 9% and this may represent a significant contribution to the change in signal intensity in a voxel. At the present time, no procedures exist for correcting the signal decay for volumetric changes in actual heterogeneous food systems. Any effects due to component density changes would be difficult to determine in multicomponent systems such as foods. A potential approach is to use the change in the lineshape intensity of another noncrystallizing component to estimate the change in volume.

MRI versus Localized Spectroscopy

During the crystallization of a component, MRI and localized spectra provide essentially the same information. The MRI signal in each voxel is proportional to the number density of mobile protons from all components. If the temperature of the phase transition for each component is distinctly different, the rate of crystallization can be determined directly from the decrease in the signal intensity in each voxel. If, however, two components are undergoing phase transitions at the same time, the decrease in signal intensity is proportional to the combined crystallization processes.

The primary advantage of using localized spectra for quantifying crystallization is that each component's transition is measured from separate signals (as shown in Fig. 5.5), and the amount of data to be analyzed is often significantly reduced (Simoneau et al. 1991).

Lipid Crystallization

Phase Volume

Low-resolution

Low-resolution spectrometers such as the Bruker Minispec® are used extensively in the food industry to measure the solid-liquid ratio of fats. These values are important for the control of processes, for quality assurance, and for development of new products. A typical experiment proceeds as follows:

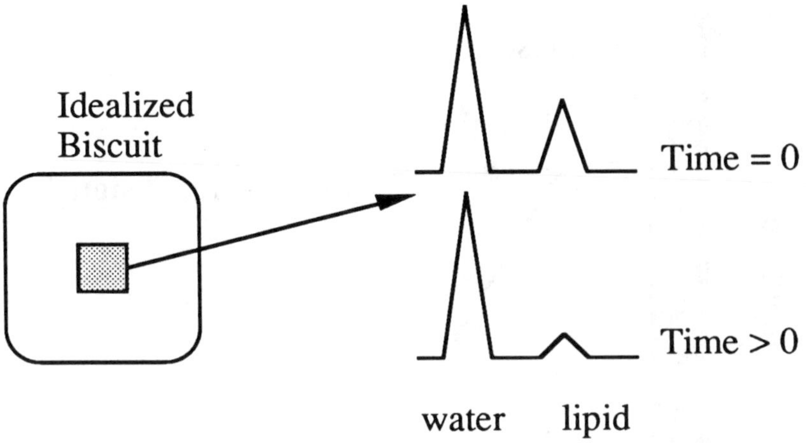

Figure 5.5. Idealized spatially resolved NMR signal from a biscuit demonstrating the changes following lipid crystallization.

1. Sample is heated until all fat is liquid.
2. Free induction decays are measured as the temperature of the sample is reduced.
3. Free induction decays are analyzed.

The analysis is performed by ratioing signal intensity values from the free induction decay, separated by a time delay. This time delay allows all solid signals to decay to zero and is thus characteristic of the amount of liquid fat. In principle, this technique appears simple. However, the greatest source of error in the technique is related to the delay time between the excitation pulse and the beginning of data acquisition. As shown in Figure 5.6, the solid signal decays during this time, and this situation requires that a correction factor be added to the solid-liquid ratio:

$$\frac{S}{L} = \frac{\text{solid signal} + \text{correction}}{\text{solid signal} + \text{correction} + \text{liquid signal}}$$

This technique has proven to be a useful quality assurance test. Moreover, the test provides information on the role of fats in product stability, texture development, and organoleptic attributes such as flavor release.

The method described in the previous paragraph is the direct method to determine the solid/liquid ratio. Other NMR methods are referred to as indirect, solid echo, and curve deconvolution (Gribnau 1992).

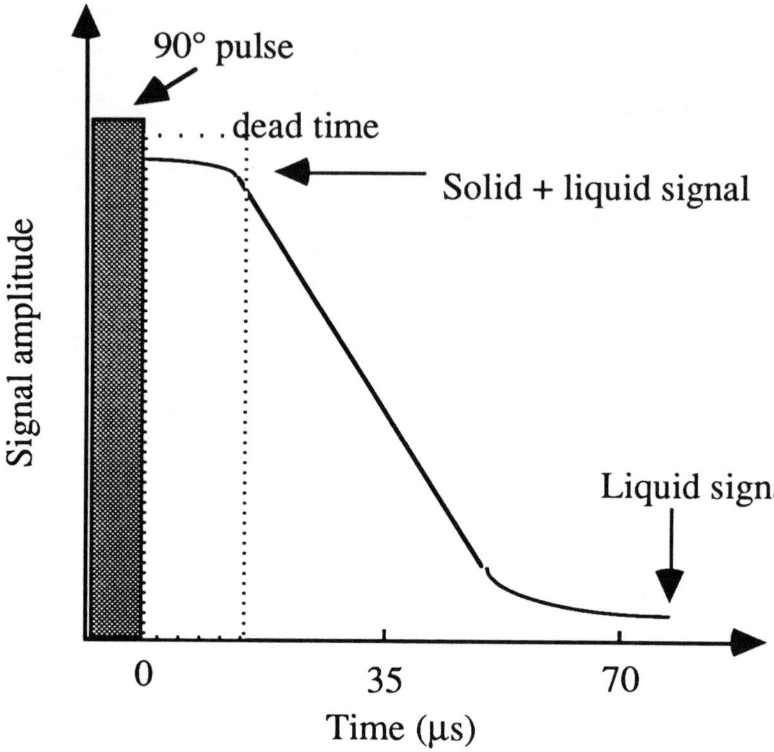

Figure 5.6. Low-resolution NMR signal decay of the solid and liquid signal from a partially frozen sample.

NMR Imaging

Spatially resolving the lipid signal has allowed for the determination of lipid crystallization rates in bulk, in model food systems, in emulsions, and in actual food systems (Duce, Carpenter & Hall 1990; Simoneau et al. 1991, 1993; McCarthy et al. 1991). The advantage of the MRI approach is that the entire sample is viewed at once and additional information such as the distribution of voids is obtained. The procedure to quantify the rate of crystallization is essentially the same as for the indirect method in low-resolution NMR experiments. The decrease in liquid signal intensity is recorded as a function of time. The difference between the signal at any time and the original signal strength is proportional to the amount of crystalline material formed.

The primary information obtained from MRI studies of lipid crystallization is the rate of crystal growth. This observed crystal growth has been modeled as having "nucleation" and "crystal growth" phases (Özilgen et al. 1993). However, these terms refer to expressions in an empirical model and should not be considered to relate to actual crystal growth and nucleation processes until a relationship is established (if indeed one exists). The parameters in the empirical model parameters may be related to the nucleation and crystal growth; however, the conditions for the phase change in bulk samples are significantly different than in a DSC. The relationship of the actual events to the observed signal decrease is an active area of investigation.

Differential Scanning Calorimetry (DSC)

DSC is an important tool for the study of crystallization phenomena. DSC is based on measuring the difference in the heat flow rate between a sample and a reference cell. The DSC measures the heat flow into or out of the sample in comparison to a reference in which no thermal events occur. For example, the heat evolution and temperature dependence of the heat evolution can be used to measure the polymorphs present in a mixture of lipids. DSC is the primary experimental technique that has been used to date for measuring the rate of solid-liquid or liquid-solid phase transition. DSC is an essential tool to use in combination with MRI when studying crystallization.

The importance of this combination was demonstrated in the study by Duce, Carpenter, and Hall (1990) on cocoa butter crystallization in chocolate. Two identical samples of chocolate were subjected to different cooling rates, one rapid and one slow. Since cooling rates can be used to promote the formation of one crystal form, the samples were expected to have different polymorphs. Differences in signal intensity existed between the two samples and were confirmed with DSC to be a result of different solid/liquid ratios of the cocoa butter, and hence the formation of distinct polymorphs. As discussed by Duce, Carpenter, and Hall (1990), care must be taken when applying this to other samples because cocoa butter is a natural fat which is a mixture of different triglyceride components and other samples may have a different total amount of lipid.

Freezing of Water

Visualization and quantification of the freezing of moisture in food allows for the optimization of freezing processes and of the formulation of frozen foods. Preliminary studies of freezing and thawing of foods have demonstrated the potential for optimizing the freezing process (McCarthy, Reid & Kauten 1994; Reid & McCarthy 1991; McCarthy et al. 1991; Fyfe et al. 1990).

Food Systems

The process of freezing has been observed in a variety of vegetables, meats, and fish in the author's laboratory (see Table 5.1). These items typically freeze in the manner illustrated in Figure 5.3. The ice interface is not a distinct region,

Table 5.1. Foods in which the freezing interface is easily observed with MRI.

Meat and Fish	Vegetables and Fruit
salmon	pears
pork	peas
beef	potatoes
chicken	corn
processed meats	onions
	carrots

but rather extends over a small length, usually at least several hundred microns and up to about a centimeter. This occurs because the freezing point of the solution in real foods changes as water is frozen and the solution becomes more concentrated in solutes. This increased concentration of solutes lowers the freezing point and hence results in a spreading of the interface into a zone over which most of the ice formation occurs.

Comparison of MRI Data to Mathematical Models

Comparing MRI data and mathematical model predictions must be done on a case-by-case basis. This is because the MRI data frequently provides details of information not accounted for in the model. For example, most models of the freezing process in foods assume a well-defined freezing temperature, and hence a well-defined ice interface should exist. However, the MRI data demonstrates that the freezing occurs over a range of temperatures and the ice interface is more appropriately described as a region of dramatic change in the liquid water signal intensity. Thus, the model and the MRI data can be approximately compared but not precisely compared.

Özilgen et al. (1994) used an enthalpy-based model for the case of freezing of a piece of beef in a simulated air-blast freezer (Mannapperuma & Singh 1988, 1989). The model was used to predict the temperature distribution in the sample and the total enthalpy removal. The enthalpy was estimated from the MRI data by taking the midpoint of the region with rapidly changing signal intensity as the ice interface. These enthalpy estimates were compared with calorimetry and model predictions and all three closely agreed. However, it should be noted that there was one adjustable parameter used in the comparison, namely, the surface heat transfer coefficient from the air to the sample. While the surface heat transfer coefficients needed to achieve agreement were within the range expected for the system, the actual measurement of the heat transfer coefficient would provide for a more stringent test.

State of Water in Frozen Systems

Using NMR to observe unfrozen moisture at very low temperatures has raised the question of how the state of the water can be described. Harz, Weisser, and

Liebenspacher (1989) have described it as kinetically inhibited from crystallizing. This inhibition arises from the increase in viscosity of the solution at low temperature and high solute concentration. The crystallization of several model systems with unfrozen water was studied over many weeks. The authors noted that after 22 weeks the glucose sample was almost totally solidified; however, the sucrose and fructose solutions remained unchanged for 35 weeks. No changes in the fructose solution were expected since the storage temperature was above that necessary for crystallization. The sucrose solution most likely needed more than 35 weeks for crystallization to occur.

References

Duce, S. L., Carpenter, T. A., & Hall, L. D. 1990. Nuclear magnetic resonance imaging of chocolate confectionery and the spatial detection of polymorphic states of cocoa butter in chocolate. *Lebensmittel-Wissenschaft und-Technologie* **23**: 565–569.

Fyfe, C. A., Burlinson, N. E., Kao, P., & Isbell, S. 1990. Nuclear magnetic resonance imaging of freezing/thawing phenomena of liquids in heterogeneous systems. In *Conference Proceedings: 31st Experimental Nuclear Magnetic Resonance Spectroscopy Conference* (p. 56). April 1–5, Asilomar Conference Center, Pacific Grove, CA.

Gribnau, M. C. M. 1992. Determination of solid/liquid ratios of fats and oils by low-resolution NMR. *Trends in Food Science and Technology* **3**: 186–190.

Harz, H.-P., Weisser, H., & Liebenspacher, F. 1989 (July). Determination of the solid/liquid ratio of frozen food by nuclear magnetic resonance (NMR) spectroscopy. In *Proceedings, International Conference on Technical Innovations in Freezing and Refrigeration of Fruits and Vegetables*, edited by D. S. Reid, 129–135. Dept. of Food Science and Technology, University of California, Davis.

Mannapperuma, J. D., & Singh, R. P. 1988. Prediction of freezing and thawing times of foods using a numerical method based on enthalpy formulation. J. *Food Science* **53**: 626–630.

Mannapperuma, J. D., & Singh, R. P. 1989. A computer aided method for the prediction of properties and freezing/thawing times of food. *J. Food Engineering* **9**: 275–304.

McCarthy, M. J., Charoenrein, S., German, J. B., McCarthy, K. L., & Reid, D. S. 1991. Phase volume measurements using magnetic resonance imaging. In *Water Relationships in Foods: Advances in the 1980s and Trends for the 1990s*, edited by H. Levine and L. Slade, 615–626. New York: Plenum Press.

McCarthy, M. J., Reid, D. S., & Kauten, R. J. 1994. Real time monitoring of the extent of freezing and thawing in foods. in press. In *Proceedings of the Symposium on Freezing,* 8th World Congress of Food Science and Technology. London: Blackie Academic and Professional.

Özilgen, S., Simoneau, C., McCarthy, M. J., German, J. B., & Reid, D. S. Crystallization kinetics of emulsified triglycerides. *J. of the Science of Food and Agriculture* **61**: 101–08.

Özilgen, M., McCarthy, M. J., Kerr, W., Kauten, R. J. and Reid, D. S. 1994. Comparison of NMR imaging and mathermatical modeling of freezing. *J. of Food Process Engineering,* in press.

Reid, D. S. & McCarthy, M. J. 1991. Magnetic resonance imaging of the process of freezing and thawing in bulk tissues, 1946, In *Proceedings of the XVIIth International Congress of Refrigeration,* **IV**, Inter. Institute of Refrigeration, Paris.

Simoneau, C., McCarthy, M. J., Kauten, R. J., & German, J. B. 1991. Crystallization dynamics in model emulsions from magnetic resonance imaging. *J. of the American Oil Chemists' Society* **68**: 481–487.

Simoneau, C., McCarthy, M. J., Reid, D. S., & German, J. B. 1993. Influence of triglyceride composition on crystallization kinetics of model emulsions. *J. of Food Engineering*. **19**: 365–387.

6

Future Trends and Conclusions

Future Trends

Applications of MRI to study foods and food processing will continue to increase as more reasonably priced MRI spectrometers become available. This should expand applications beyond those contained or suggested in this book. Developments in both the hardware and the software used in magnetic resonance imaging are proceeding at a rapid pace and should act to catalyze new applications. The major trends in MRI from the field of medicine will probably be transferred to other fields, including food science. Wehrli (1992) recently summarized the major trends in medical MRI as follows:

1. Development of ultrafast imaging procedures
2. Incorporation of expert systems
3. Enhancement of chemical shift imaging of nuclei with low NMR sensitivity (C-13, Na-23)

Improvements in the speed of acquiring MRI data will help in studying fast processes such as roasting, rapid freezing, mixing, and extrusion. Incorporating expert systems will increase the likelihood of on-line MRI sensors for use in process control. The expert system should allow control of a process with limited MRI data. Improvements in chemical shift imaging will be especially useful for understanding the role of salt and macromolecules in food systems.

In addition to these trends, the author expects that q-space imaging will become an important technique. *q-space imaging* is the term used to describe the procedure employed to determine the translational displacement probability. This allows measurement not only of the diffusion coefficient but also of pore spacing and mean pore size (Callaghan 1991; Callaghan et al. 1991; Cotts 1991). As an analog to q-space imaging, Maneval and McCarthy (1992) have recently used p-space imaging where p is the Fourier conjugate variable for velocity. P-space imaging can be used to measure structural features such as pore size distributions.

These developments will, in turn, probably have an impact on two areas of food science, analytical methods and process control sensors.

Analytical Methods

MRI provides information on food structure, phase transitions, rheology, and component functionality. This information is most often complementary to information provided by existing experimental methods. For example, NMR and DSC are good experimental techniques to use in combination for studies of crystallization phenomena in foods (as presented in Chapter 5). Advances in microscopic MRI and imaging of low NMR sensitivity nuclei should become more prevalent. Microscopic MRI will prove useful in studying the development of food structure at length scales between MRI and electron microscopy. The imaging of nuclei with low NMR sensitivity such as C-13 or Na-23 should be useful for studying reactions involving macromolecules, phase transitions of sugars, and diffusion of salt.

Process Control Sensor

As food producers strive to meet increasingly high quality standards and government labeling requirements, new process control sensors are needed. NMR and MRI are potentially good methods for monitoring a number of quality attributes or process parameters. The advantages of NMR-based sensors are primarily that they are noninvasive and nondestructive. They hold the potential to make measurements without disturbing the process or introducing potential contaminants such as chemicals or glass into a process stream. Additionally, NMR signals are sensitive to motion and could make good on-line rheometers. Potential applications include control of food freezing, aseptic processing, and in-package quality control.

The additional technical difficulties involved with placing NMR on-line are related to the magnet shape and the speed of data acquisition. Recent advances in magnet design indicate that several new configurations may be viable. One example would be using a superconducting magnet together with a permanent magnet to achieve a uniform field on a conveyor. An alternate approach would be to use a pulsed magnetic field and perform the NMR experiment at zero field or in the earth's magnetic field.

Speed of MRI data acquisition has been significantly improved in recent years. Information that formerly required minutes to acquire can now be gotten in tens of milliseconds. Additionally, several food samples can be analyzed simultaneously by the same sensor, which results in a significant increase in throughput. This information can be acquired from moving samples or from groups of moving

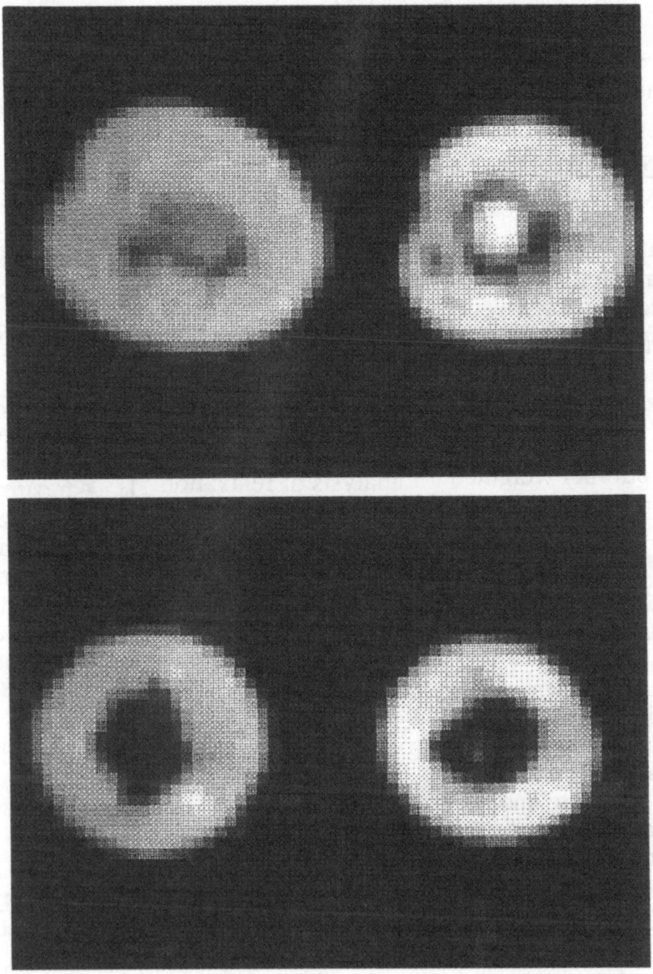

Figure 6.1. Two-dimensional hydrogen NMR spin echo images of cherries with and without pits.

samples. For example, the pits in cherries can be detected by simple 2-D or 1-D MR images; the 2-D images are shown in Figure 6.1.

Conclusions

MRI is an excellent experimental tool for characterizing the physical properties, structure, and transport properties of biological materials. The utility of this experimental technique is summarized in Figure 6.2. This outline serves as a

FOOD STRUCTURE

Moisture, void & lipid distributions	Emulsions & foams	Suspensions
Relaxation weighted imaging • for spatial distribution of water and lipid and other structural features Chemical shift imaging • to quantify the spatial concentration of each phase Susceptibility weighted imaging • to determine the distribution & approximate volume of voids Diffusion weighted imaging • to determine the quantity & spatial distribution of each phase • to obtain information on the structure and permeability of membranes	*VOLUME FRACTIONS* Chemical shift imaging or relaxation weighted imaging *PARTICLE SIZE* PGSE NMR or analysis of relaxation decay curves	*VELOCITY PROFILES* Phase encoded or time-of-flight *RHEOLOGICAL INFORMATION* From analysis of velocity profiles one can obtain • apparent yield stress • constituitive model parameters • particle concentrations and distributions

Figure 6.2. Summary of approaches to measure food structure using MRI.

summary of applications discussed in this book and as a starting point for food scientists and food engineers interested in applying MRI to food structure measurement. The applications of MRI in the study of food and biological materials will continue to expand. The expansion of the applications will most likely occur first in analytical applications and eventually in process control situations. In addition to the applications discussed, the development of solid-state magnetic resonance imaging methods will permit the examination of large molecules in an imaging mode. The development and use of solid-state imaging protocols should be one of the most active areas of research in the future.

References

Callaghan, P. T. 1991. *Principles of Nuclear Magnetic Resonance Microscopy*. New York: Oxford University Press.

Callaghan, P. T., Coy A., MacGowan, D., Packer, K. J., & Zelaya, F. O. 1991. Diffraction-like effects in NMR diffusion studies of fluids in porous solids. *Nature* **351**: 467–469.

Cotts, R. M. 1991. NMR—Diffusion and diffraction. *Nature* **351**: 443–444.

Maneval, J. E., & McCarthy, M. J. 1992 (June). NMR flow measurements in porous media: The role of th microstructure. Paper presented at the Workshop in NMR Imaging, 66th Colloid Conference, American Chemical Society, Morgantown, West Virginia.

Wehrli, F. W. 1992. The origins and future of nuclear magnetic resonance imaging. *Physics Today* **45**: 34–42.

Index

Agricultural products (*see also* Foods)
animals 84
time scale in measuring drying 52
Air bubbles 23, 24, 56
Air pockets (*see* Voids)
Analysis of NMR signal
dynamics 52
flow measurements 52–54
MRI versus localized spectroscopy 94
phase volume changes 94
phase volume measurements & concentrations 51–52
quantification of water & lipid signals 74–75
relaxation effects 72–74, 90–91
spin-warp imaging 72
temperature effects 74, 91–93
Apples 78, 79
Artifacts 25, 49

Beans, dry 17
Beer 52, 58
Biscuits 56, 57, 59, 84, 95
Bubbles (*see* Voids)

Cakes 56
Carrot 21
Cheese
curd shrinkage & whey migration 17
internal structure 1–3
oil/water distribution 14
Cherries 103
Chocolate 84, 97
Conversion of measurements 75–78
Cookies 56
Corn 80
Crystallization 94, 96, 97, 99 (*see also* Freezing)

Differential scanning calorimetry 97
Drying
agricultural materials 52
apples 17, 78, 79
corn 17, 80
porous media 80–83
potatoes 78–79
rate curve 82, 83
DSC (*see* Differential scanning calorimetry)

Eggs 57, 61
Egg white 57
Electron paramagnetic resonance 4
Electron spin resonance 4
Emulsions 16–17, 57–61, 96, 104
ESR (*see* Electron spin resonance)
Experimental setup
changing sample 91
designing & building equipment 48–49, 88–89
during freezing 88–89
during lipid crystallization 94–95
in general 5–14, 33–37, 38–41
to measure food structure 45–51
foams 54–56
emulsions 57–61
suspensions 62–67
to measure moisture & lipid distribution 70–72
to measure phase transitions 88–89

Fat (*see* Lipids)
Film thickness measurements 82–83
Fish 25, 98
Foams 14–16, 45, 52, 54–57, 58, 104
Food research (*see also* Rheology)
  applications & impact of MRI on 14–21, 102–103
  future trends 101–103
  MRI component functionality in 45–67
  MRI provides complementary information to existing methods 102
  on live animals 84
  processed food 84–86
Foods
  apples 78
  beans, dry 17
  beefsteak 92
  beer 52
  biscuits 56, 57, 59, 84, 95
  cakes 56
  carrot 21
  cheese 1–3, 14, 17
  cherries 103
  chocolate 84, 97
  cookies 56
  corn 80
  eggs 57, 61
  egg white 57
  fish 25
  fruit juices 62
  ice cream 57
  liver, goose 84
  oil 14
  peanut butter 84
  potatoes 78–79, 85
  salad dressings 14
  soups & stews 62
  tomato juice 1–3, 62
Food stability and structure
  emulsions 16–17
  freezing 97–98
  foams 14–16
  gels 17
  measurement of moisture & lipid distribution 70–86
    saturation 70–78
    moisture saturation 78–83
    lipid saturation 83–86
  measurement of structure 45–54
    emulsions 57–61
    foams 54–57
    gels 17
    suspensions 61–67
  moisture migration 17–18
    dehydration/rehydration 17–18
    storage 18–19
  phase changes 19–21
    freezing 19–20
    lipid crystallization 20–21
  rheology 19
  summary of methods to measure food structure 104
Food structure (*see* Food stability and structure)
Freezing
  beef 92, 98
  carrot 21
  comparison of MRI data to mathematical models 98
  correction of freezing curve 93
  foods in which freezing interface is easily observed 98
  irregular-shaped food products 93
  meat and fish 97–98
  modifications to air-blast freezer 90
  movement of ice interface 19–20
  phase volume changes in water & lipids 94
  placement of probe during 88
  signal decay from partially frozen sample 96
  temperature range during 22
  vegetables and fruit 98
  water 97–99
Fructose 99
Fruit 98
Fruit juice 62

Gels 17, 23
Glucose 99

Ice cream 57
Imaging
  chemical shift 14
  comparison of data to theoretical models 42–43
  density 22
  diffusion/flow 22
  digital nature of data 23
  information content of 41–42
  MRI 37–41
    echo planar 41
    Fourier 40–41
    frequency encoding 40

phase encoding 39–40
projection reconstruction 41
slice selection 38–39
property-weighted 14
resolution of image 26–27
spin-warp 41–43, 72
structural 23
temperature 22–23

Juice
fruit 62
tomato 1–3, 62

Lipids (*see also* Oil)
crystallization 20–21, 94–97
distribution measurements 70–86, 104
fat-weighted MRI 25
migration in American-style biscuit 84–85
phase volume changes 94
quantification of signals 74–75
relationship of signal intensities to concentration values 75–78
saturation measurements 70–78, 83–86
structural imaging of 23–24

Magnetic resonance imaging (*see* MRI)
Measurement
conversions 75–78
film thickness 82–83
influence of different feed formulations on animals 84
lipids in goose liver 84
muscle structure of animals 84
Meat 92, 98
Medical use of NMR/MRI 5, 6, 84
Moisture distribution
in American-style biscuit 84–85
moisture profile of drying apple 79
relationship of signal intensities to concentration 75–78
saturation measurements 78–83
Moisture migration
dehydration/rehydration 17–18
storage 18–19
MRI
animal feeding & breeding uses 84
applications & impact on food research 14–21
capabilities & limitations 21–27
characteristics of 4
comparison of data to mathematical models 98
definition of 3
echo planar imaging 41
Fourier imaging 40–41
frequency encoding 40
fundamental principles of 30–43
future trends in usage 101–103
history of NMR 4–5
introduction to 3
medical uses of 5, 84
multiple uses of 5
phase encoding 39–40
processed food analysis 84–86
projection reconstruction 41
slice selection 38–39
techniques 11–14
property-weighted imaging 14
chemical shift imaging 14
microscopy 14
versus localized spectroscopy 94
Moisture saturation measurements 78–83

NMR
analysis of signal 51–54, 72–75, 90–94
basis of theoretical models 42–43
Bloch model of 31–33
characteristics of 4
comparison of image data to theoretical models 42–43
definition of 3–4
diagram of NMR spectrum 8
diagram of time domain signal from sample in low-resolution spectrometer 9
equipment & experiments 5–14
high-resolution 7–8
history of 4–5
information content of image 41–42
low-resolution 7–8
mathematical basis for comparison of image data to theoretical models 43
medical use of 5
medical terminology 3
multiple uses of 5
pulsed field gradient experiments 10–11
pulse sequences 7
quantum mechanical description 30–31
spectrometer components 5–7
spectrum 7–8
use of high-resolution 10
NMR equipment and experiments 5–14

components of spectrometer 5–7
designing & building 48–49
high-resolution 10
low-resolution 7–8
pulsed field gradient experiments 10–11
pulse sequences 7
two-dimensional 10
Nuclear magnetic resonance (*see* NMR)

Oil (*see also* Lipids)
distribution determined by chemical shift imaging 14
oil/water interface 25
profile of oil on top of water 26

Peanut butter 84
Phase transitions 19–20, 20–21, 88–99
Potatoes 78–79, 85
Probe
birdcage coil 47, 71
diagram of birdcage & surface coils 47
diagram of solenoid coil 6
diagram of probe configuration for precise sample placement 73
different designs for 7, 45–47
Pulse sequences
one-pulse 33–34
spin echo 34–37
stimulated echo 37

Rehydration, potatoes & dry beans 17
Rheology 19, 52–54, 62–67, 102, 104

Salad dressings
chemical shift imaging to determine oil/water distribution 14
quantification of amount of oil 85
Sample
best shapes 71–72
container 46–47, 71–72, 88–89
placement within probe 73
system for changing 91

Sensor
use to study freezing 19–20
Setup (*see* Experimental setup)
Shielded gradients 50–51
Signal-to-noise ratio 45, 70–71, 88
Soups, vegetable 62
Spectrometer
component functionality 45–67
components of 5–7
diagram of 6
setup 45, 49–50, 72, 89
Spin-warp imaging signals 41–43
Stews 62
Structure
emulsions 57–61
foams 54–57
gels 17, 23
measurement of food 45–67
suspensions 61–67
water frozen in food 97–99
Sucrose
high-resolution NMR spectrum of hydrogen in 11
low temperature state 99
two-dimensional NMR spectrum of hydrogen in 11
Suspensions 61–67, 104

Techniques of MRI 14
Tomato juice 1–3, 62

Vegetables 98
Voids 23, 56, 84, 104
Voxel 23, 26, 42, 55, 72, 79, 94

Water
distribution determined by chemical shift imaging 14
freezing in food systems 97–98
freezing of 97–99
oil/water interface 25
profile of oil on top of water 26
quantification of signals 74–75
state in frozen systems 98–99
structural imaging of 23–24